PRAISE FOR DR. PAUL

At age 55, I began a march from a La-Z-Boy lifestyle to a 2011 gold medal-winning National Cycling Championship podium. In two short years, Dr. Paul helped me achieve what seemed to everyone around me to be impossible.

— *Bill Watkins, world-class athlete, founder of The Lions Pride*

Dr. Paul masterfully guides the reader through a maze of diets and exercise programs. He navigates through current complex and sometimes conflicting research on nutrition and exercise and designs a simple, yet comprehensive evidence-based program with his passionate prose.

— *Gaetano J. Scuderi, MD, certified orthopedic spine surgeon, professor, Stanford University*

This book will be instrumental in creating a health and fitness movement that we have not yet experienced in this century.

— *David T.S. Wood, speaker, trainer, and philanthropist*

Dr. Paul's Protein Pacing Diet eloquently combines his outstanding scientific acumen and passion for us all to lead fulfilling and meaningful lives by successfully optimizing human performance, health, and relationships.

— *Meghan Downs, Ph.D., NASA physiologist*

"Protein Pacing and The PRISE Life Protocol answers all our needs to stay in shape. Dr. Paul helps us understand how our bodies work the most efficiently and keep us fit for what he calls this 'race of life.' Dr. Paul is a remarkable resource for the sports science community."

— *Amy Peterson, USA short track speed skating, five-time Olympian*

"Dr. Paul Arciero's PRISE Life is truly the way to a healthy lifestyle, better performance, and a happier life."

— *Brad Faxon, PGA champion*

THE PRISE LIFE®

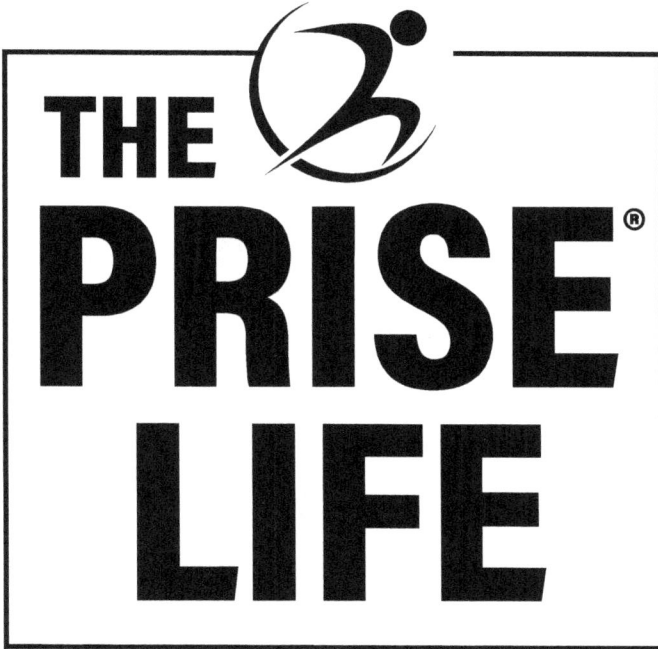

Protein Pacing
for Optimal Health
and Performance

THE PRISE® LIFE

Protein Pacing for Optimal Health and Performance

DR. PAUL J. ARCIERO

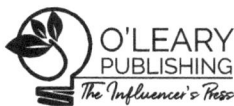

O'LEARY
PUBLISHING
The Influencer's Press

BONITA SPRINGS, FL

To get 7 Free Protein Pacing Recipes visit www.priselife.com
For wholesale pricing please email: info@olearypublishing.com
This book is not intended as a substitute for the medical advice of
physicians. The reader should regularly consult a physician in matters
relating to his/her health and particularly with respect to any symptoms
that may require diagnosis or medical attention.

ISBN 978-1-7341589-3-9 (print)
ISBN 978-1-7341589-4-6 (ebook)
Library of Congress Control Number 2019917621

Design by Jessica Angerstein
Photography by Louis Venne Photography
Edited by Heather Davis Desrocher
Line Editing by Gregory Schriver
Editorial Support by Wilson Hawthorne

Printed in the United States of America

This book is dedicated to my grandparents:
John Petrillo and Edith "Deedie" Arciero.

And to my parents: Donald Vincent Arciero
and Jane Barbara (Petrillo) Arciero.

This book is also for you, my dedicated and
ever-growing tribe of supporters, now reaching into the
millions. Everything in this book links back to
what you have graciously taught me along the way.

Your devotion, which helped me to commit to the
scientific process, has led to a well-documented and scientifically-
proven roadmap to achieving optimal health and peak performance.
The PRISE Life and Protein Pacing are now yours to attain.

Above all, know that I am committed to you finding a deep love of
yourself, a gift that in return will honor you with a truly fulfilling
and meaningful life—the kind that I have been so blessed to find.

CONTENTS

FOREWORD

Principles. Universal truths.

Enduring foundations on which the world operates.

My late father, Dr. Stephen R. Covey, studied, practiced, and taught the principles of leadership and effectiveness throughout his life. I've followed his example in seeking to deeply understand and share the lasting principles upon which trusting relationships, organizations, and societies are built and prosper. Now Dr. Paul Arciero has done the same with the enduring principles that ensure human health, fitness, and performance. What a wonderful contribution this is!

I'll never forget the day I met Dr. Paul. We were both speaking at a conference several years ago when we first conversed, and later that day, while at the airport as we prepared to head to our next destinations, we had another discussion. I found Paul to be a credible and trusted source for the principles and practices of health and fitness, and equally important, a sincere and genuine individual driven by a mission in life to help people optimize their health and happiness.

In Western societies, we are struggling with epidemic levels of obesity, diabetes, heart disease, cancers, and many new lifestyle-related diseases. They are rapidly increasing because people are unaware, misinformed, or ignoring the basic principles of wise eating, exercise, and energy management. That's where Dr. Paul's work comes in. Backed by scientific data and peer-reviewed research, Dr. Paul lays out the principles that underlie health and fitness in a way that challenges our age-old assumptions and shifts our paradigms.

As you study this marvelous book, you will gain greater understanding, and motivation to practice the principles of health and vitality that Paul calls The PRISE Life Protocol. Fad diets and body-punishing exercise regimes are much like the get-rich-quick, pop psychology advice you see in hundreds of books and websites. By contrast, the principles that undergird PRISE are sound, based on peer-reviewed research, then published in credible scientific journals. This is not a get-fit-quick solution. It's a solid, beneficial program of resistance, high-intensity interval, stretching, and endurance training, proper eating, and sleep that, if followed, will deliver on its promise.

For example, Dr. Paul breaks ground on what pacing your protein really means—how he created it, how the timing of what you eat is critical, and how much of what types of food you eat can literally change your life. He teaches us the value of high-quality nourishment and fitness training to improve energy metabolism, body composition, and glucose tolerance; how to lessen the risk of cardiovascular disease by losing adipose tissue (especially belly fat); and how to gain more control over our body and health.

But don't worry, with the empirical data to back up his PRISE Life Protocol, Dr. Paul makes this an easy-to-read book, reminding us about macros (those proteins, fats, and carbohydrates), and then simplifies everything with easy-to-follow charts. You can finally achieve the optimal health and fitness you have always dreamed about and might even be able to push yourself to peak performance levels that you had long given up on.

This is a very current and important piece of work. Dr. Paul shows that although a healthy lifestyle takes commitment, nutrition and exercise don't need to be as complicated as we are being led by the hype to believe.

Of course, a healthy lifestyle incorporates exercise, but it is amazing how much easier movement is when we feel good or don't have such extreme time- and energy-expending hurdles to overcome. He demonstrates how energy is our life's force and how ultimately we want the same thing: health and longevity to spend quality time doing what we love with and for our loved ones. To me, this works for us folks with busy work schedules, all the way to Olympians and star athletes. Dr. Paul knows—he was a tennis champion himself and shares his struggles and journeys in a wonderful heartfelt chapter.

I've validated these principles myself through years of struggling with my weight fluctuating up and down (mostly going up) as I've attempted to manage constant global travel, meals on the run, and a jam-packed schedule as an executive and now as a professional speaker and author. Even though I have a discipline of exercising at least thirty minutes every day, I've learned several new strategies and approaches in this book that I'm confident will take me to the next level of fitness and performance.

Perhaps what has been most inspirational to me in Dr. Paul's book is his explanation of who trusted him. I loved reading how he found his voice as a young person and pursued that passion through his academic studies, as a competitive athlete, and as a gifted human being. And how did he find his voice? Through the encouragement and support of loved ones, especially "Grandma Deedie," "Grandpa," "Big D," his dad, and his mother, the "85-year-old hiking grandmother." I love to hear, collect, and share the stories of how people respond when they're trusted, and I believe you will be inspired as you read Dr. Paul's and enjoy the results from applying the teachings of this book.

Thank you, Paul, for your wonderful work and for the pleasure it gives me to see how you have focused on principles in the health and fitness dimension, much like my father and I have focused on principles in the human and organizational effectiveness dimension. Seeing a parallel focus around universal principles is what continues to make my life infinitely rewarding.

I look forward to our next chance encounter on the speaking circuit or even at an airport!

Stephen M. R. Covey

Author of the *New York Times* and the *Wall Street Journal* best-selling book, *The Speed of Trust,* former president and CEO of Covey Leadership Center

INTRODUCTION

Let me begin by sharing that I am going to take you on a journey—a journey about what a healthy lifestyle really means. All of us have a journey, and this is mine. My goal is to help you live your journey with more health and with better nutrition, fitness, and performance. This is not a regular diet and fitness book. This book is the culmination of over thirty years of research and the deep belief that science mimics the perfection of nature and that if we follow its rules, the way we were originally created (which may be simpler than you believe), we can all achieve optimal health and fitness, and even longevity.

I understand this is a bold statement in a world where we want things to be quick and inexpensive. I am here to tell you that after more than thirty years of research as a scientist, as well as an athlete, coach, and consultant, I've studied and dissected all these up-and-coming ideas and discovered there is an actual roadmap, protocol, recipe, and, in fact, key, to finding and achieving health. It is no longer a mystery, and it absolutely does not have to cost you a fortune. Throughout this book, I share the science behind The PRISE Life Protocol, including the discovery of Protein Pacing. And I provide peer-reviewed material, with proven science, to establish even more credibility for The PRISE Life and Protein Pacing.

I will guide you through the simple steps that evolved from my personal struggle to stay healthy and fit in a stressful world where we find ourselves short of time. You will hear the stories that fueled my passion to help others be healthy. I will show that you, too, can "Keep Your Eyes on The PRISE" and finally claim the ultimate weight, health, and longevity you deserve. I will introduce you to the application of Protein Pacing and The PRISE Protocol so you can seamlessly and synergistically incorporate these into your own life to give you the best results you've ever seen.

With my research devoted to human performance, nutrition, and applied physiology, as well as neuropsychology and cognitive development, I have discovered a fascinating understanding of how the human body functions best, the way nature intended it to be— without overexertion, dehydration, crazy 500 calorie-a-day diets, injections, steroids, medications, bypass surgeries, sugar-packed meal replacement powders and bars, stimulants, deprivation, overanalyzing, and so on.

I will share with you groundbreaking studies from the relatively new and exciting fields of human performance, nutrition, neuroscience, and applied physiology. According to the American College of Sports Medicine (ACSM), the leading and most respected authority on sports medicine and related fields, "Nutrition for sport is the provision of essential nutrients, including fuels and fluids, to provide energy for training, competition, recovery, and general health and wellness. The intake versus expenditure of these essential nutrients will be called energy balance. Optimum performance is promoted by adequate energy intake."

This is exactly what I do when I research what foods to eat when, in what quantity, how much fluid is needed, and how this pertains to either recovery or greater wellness in my subjects. We need the energy to live, and there is an actual method of getting the proper nutrition to support the human body.

As for achieving health, isn't the core of life about the nutrition part of eating right, getting the proper fluids into the body, and then exercising properly? I know the commonly held belief is that to maintain a healthy lifestyle you must eat less and exercise more. But my message is nearly the opposite of this... I am going to show you a way to eat more high-quality foods and pay less attention to the quantity of food you eat, and then how to exercise smarter, not harder and longer. So hold on, hold on, I will get there!

As a nutrition and applied physiology scientist, I'm interested in the interaction between environmental factors, nutrition, exercise, and disease on human function, as well as the physiological mechanisms regulating human health and performance. I work to understand how to reverse disease progression and how to encourage peak physical performance, always working from the level the person is currently at to safely increase their results. Aren't we seeking ways that, with proper nutrition and exercise, we can work to attain optimal health, perhaps even sustained peak performance, and reverse disease all for the goal of living a long and healthy life? Or, in simpler terms, aren't we just working to look and feel better?

In the past, I've been the scientist hidden in the lab, but now I am here to share my research with you. This journey of life can lead to bettering humankind or hindering the future of our planet and our lives. Which path do you choose? I'm hoping that with the information I share in this book, you will find the motivation to throw away all those crazy temporary diet ideas and exercise fads and follow my roadmap of The PRISE Life Protocol with Protein Pacing and choose optimal health and peak performance!

Dr. Paul Arciero

P.S. Make sure you download The PRISE Life app today to get started.

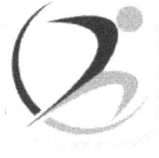

DOWNLOAD THE PRISE® LIFE APP NOW!

This is an interactive book. We have made it that way so you can have a holistic and healthy lifestyle experience. Please download The PRISE Life app from the App Store or Google Play store FREE.

Here's why!

Developed by Dr. Paul Arciero, The PRISE Life app is a novel approach to personalized nutrition, fitness, and emotional well-being. The underlying algorithms are based on Dr. Paul's thirty years of research and his groundbreaking discovery of The PRISE Protocol and Protein Pacing.

The PRISE Life app offers an individualized navigational tool. Put in a few key indicators and this app will guide you to the appropriate lifestyle choice to either lose weight, increase energy, or improve physical/athletic performance, with the primary goal of enhanced health, fitness, and wellness but without all the logging!

Ultimately, The PRISE LIfe app aims to drastically improve the way you achieve personal self-care, optimal health, and peak performance. It is the ultimate user experience for your personalized PRISE Life and Protein Pacing plan during the day, and will help you choose the most effective lifestyle strategy to enhance your health and performance.

The PRISE Life app is a companion tool to this book to help you create a lifestyle you can stay committed to and experience the best results ever! It is the first app of its kind. The PRISE Life app is like having Dr. Paul and PRISE with you all the time!

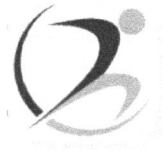

THE PRISE LIFE
PROTOCOL

CHAPTER 1
MY JOURNEY

Life is what happens to you while
you are busy making other plans.
— John Lennon

To this day, it still makes my heart sink when I realize how easy it is for people to look at others and judge. The truth is, if you heard the stories behind any person's journey, you would most likely hear about some devastating times where they were at their worst, hitting barriers that seemed utterly impossible to rise above. Rest assured, although it might not seem like it now, we all encounter these hard times along the way to finding our true selves or even our "callings." I am no stranger to struggle, and in all honesty, I have had some hard lessons and bumps along the road, too. Just like most, or all, of you.

Have they made me stronger?

Have they made me who I am today?

Of course, but they were deeply painful, and I will fully disclose my life to all of you . . . After all, it may look like I have it all together at this moment, but it hasn't always been so easy.

Here's my story.

CHILDHOOD LESSONS

I was a terrible student from the start. Teachers and administrators asked my parents to hold me back in the first grade, and then again in the fifth. To make matters worse, my first-grade teacher taught me to spell my last name wrong! Not a very good start to life. And the fact that the higher-ups decided to place me in the slower-moving classes didn't help me feel very confident about learning. Fortunately, fate intervened.

First, my mother, for whatever reason, among her seven children, had me tagging along with her to tend our two small plots at the local community garden. It was there, beginning in the sunny afternoons of spring, through the hot and muggy days of summer, and ending with the brisk days of fall, where I would spend time gardening. Just me and my mom. In the most basic sense, this experience taught me the importance of nourishing our bodies with the highest-quality food. But in a more philosophical sense, this experience of nurturing a living organism through its life cycle— beginning with a tiny seed and giving it just the right amount of water, sun, soil, and protection to support its growth and crop yield—held much more significance.

At about the same time, my dad was supporting my innate need to move my body and be physical. I started to participate in all kinds of movement experiences. I remember being introduced to a trampoline and a climbing rope in gym class, and I immediately started to push my limits on the trampoline by doing flips and twists. I caught the eye of the gym teacher and was invited to show my skill during an elementary talent show.

A LOVE FOR SPORTS

I experimented with all sorts of sports and activities, but the two that I loved most were ice hockey, no surprise there since I'm from New England, and tennis. My early childhood memories of playing youth hockey included my dad gently pulling on my toes under my bed covers at 5:00 a.m. on Saturdays to get me to outdoor hockey practice in below-freezing temperatures; it was called training, but at times felt like cruelty! I'm so grateful, my dad was always smiling and supportive on all those cold mornings and weekend-long tournaments in the wintry cold Northeast.

Through high school, my tennis game became increasingly competitive, enough to earn me a scholarship to play in college despite graduating high school in the lower quartile of about 375 students. The defining feature of my early athletic experiences were my parents always being there for me and supporting me unconditionally and without criticism or comment. I cherish the times we spent together on my journey as an athlete, because they were instrumental in building my self-confidence and self-worth, and gave me a lifelong appreciation and love of physical movement.

Ultimately, these experiences are the reason I chose a career as a nutrition and applied exercise scientist with the sole mission of helping others live a lifetime of abundant health and achieve optimal performance.

Lastly, and perhaps most impactful of my early life experiences, I had a special bond and fondness with my paternal grandmother and maternal grandfather, even among my six siblings and many other grandchildren who needed their love. Their unwavering love kept me in the game of life when I was feeling down and out.

When my grandparents, and eventually my dad's health began to fail during my teenage years, it broke me, so much so that I dedicated myself to pursue a career that could help them, and others, live healthier lives. It was the special bonds I developed with my mom, dad, and grandparents that became the core principles of how and why I live my life today and why you have this book in your hands. Without them, I wouldn't have had the courage to pursue my dreams and the confidence to overcome some of the learning challenges I faced early in my life.

HITTING ROCK BOTTOM

But along the way, I started to fight myself on everything. All of a sudden, the false foundations my psyche had been standing on all those years came crumbling down, and I could not wrap myself around my studies or sports and follow through. I was unable to deal with the idea that I could only be good if I was the best in a sport. The net result: I dropped out of college despite the fact that I had a tennis scholarship. Yes, you read those words correctly. I quit. I was so lost. I was emotional and uncommitted and confused and could not pull it together.

At the same time, my older brother and mentor, John, had recently graduated from college as an All-American tennis player and decided to compete on the European Satellite tennis tour. So, as a nineteen-year-old college dropout, I decided to join him. About seven weeks into our tennis tour experience I had barely won a match and hit rock bottom emotionally and physically. And then, the universe stepped in.

At the tournament site in Saint-Girons, France, there was a beautifully serene brook tucked away behind the tennis courts. Before the tournament started, I found myself sitting beside the brook, mesmerized by the sound of the water gently flowing over the rocks and the glitter of sunshine peeking through the treetops overhead. I remember lying down and going into what I now believe to be a state of mindfulness meditation that completely transformed my entire body. With tears streaming down, I felt I was in perfect harmony—spirit, mind, and body. In fact, it was my first experience performing what I've since referred to as the 'body visit' or 'body scan'.

A SUDDEN BREAKTHROUGH

I knew right then and there what my life was meant to be… service to others by being a resource of optimal health and peak performance. That single defining moment changed my life and set me on this journey that, decades of education and research later, I'm sharing with you in this book. Despite my horrendous performance up until this point, this harmony carried over to the tennis court, and I won the tournament and became a European tennis champion!

While I should have been gloriously celebrating, I was suddenly homesick for my parents, especially my dad. Without being able to explain it to anyone, after the most memorable athletic accomplishment in my life up to that point, I made the decision to return home the following week and re-enroll in college. Several years later, my father would be diagnosed with a very rare form of cancer and pass away at the age of sixty. I now know why I was called to come home.

RELEARNING LEARNING

My newfound commitment to education was evident. I excelled in my field of study and earned some prestigious degrees. My love for research, science, nutrition, and exercise physiology, now all seemed to make sense. Our childhood experiences really do form who we are and can show us glimpses of what we are meant to be.

I must admit that when I think of those early days and my family, even writing about it now, I get emotional. If you have ever attended one of my presentations, you have probably seen my eyes well up with tears. Part of that is natural; I'm Italian, after all. But another part is that sometimes I am astounded to be standing there sharing the material I've dedicated my life to studying. I hope that it will be the light that helps you wake up, take action, and make a change in your own life or help someone you love.

As I see my children grow and feel a deep appreciation for the love of my wife and family, I realize how strange it is to have been born into this family, at this time, with the characteristics I have been granted, both good and bad.

THE ARCHER

At some point along the way, I learned about some of my Southern Italian heritage, including my name, "Arciero," which means "archer," or "bowman," and it has become a fun exploration of how there might be something to a name. I was intrigued about the symbology and heritage behind the archer, especially when I read that an archer is born and driven to hit the mark. They have an internal, unquenchable need to take a specific area of focus and—with incredible forethought, great strength, clarity of attention, and the ability to cut out all the other noise, created internally or externally—work repeatedly for many years to get that bow and arrow to hit dead center. Now that I look back at my discoveries, in an odd sense this is exactly what I have done!

Like most discoveries, it didn't happen in a bubble. It took years of peeling the layers back to find the answer. But I don't want you to walk away with another quick discovery. I want you to walk away with a willingness, a drive, and a desire to make a personal change for the better for you and your loved ones. I know that life can be hard, and we can all be fragile at times. But if my life stories help you see that you are not the only person who has ever suffered, then perhaps the discoveries I have made will make sense and become the building blocks to a new and healthier life for all those you touch: I refer to this as "geometric growth" and the "force multiplier," or ripple effect, as some call it.

HUMAN PSYCHOLOGY

Before I get into all the specifics of my scientific breakthroughs, I want to share a little human psychology, because in the end, we are mind, body, and spirit, and to live a balanced and healthy life, we need to take all this into account. Yes, I am a scientist. I believe in defined, explained, and rational scientifically proven data, but I am also a human being who believes in the power of the mind and positive intention-based thinking. As I have evolved, I have come to embrace the spiritual components of life more and more. When combining all three, as most top achievers or happy people do, you can finally reach your dreams.

Human development combines physical growth with the psychological cycle of life. Different ages and stages of our lives present us with different tasks to conquer. With more than five-and-a-half decades to my development emotionally, physically, and spiritually, I have discovered that I am living proof of this. I am finally in that odd position where I can look back past the ups and downs of my early years and start to make sense of this science experiment called life.

When we are young, we are egocentric; we have the magical thinking of an eight-year-old. We focus on what everyone else is getting and what we are not getting. You may have had a healthy start to life with nurturing parents, or you may have had a difficult start, one defined by deprivation and neglect, leaving you frustrated, upset, hurt, or even lost. As children, we live much of our lives in the pretend world. We spend our time dreaming of better things to come because that's what we as humans do. You may dream of winning an Olympic gold medal, becoming a famous actor, winning a Nobel Peace Prize, or simply having a healthy, simple life. No matter our situations, this magical thinking stage helps us to plan our future or work through life's lessons.

THE EGO TAKES OVER

As you age, the ego takes hold, and it may or may not have your best interest in mind. You start getting trapped in the real world of hard knocks, all while trying to bring mind, body, and spirit into harmony and balance. You find yourself conflicted between your need for immediate gratification, recognition, love, and acceptance and the constant temptation of comparing yourself to others. The criticizing authoritarian in your mind jumps in. You either become an extrovert, the competitor, the one who is the best, and can be "seen," or you start to retreat into introversion. Introversion is where you find things to keep you occupied, often alone, so as to avoid others. This may simply be because you are just that uncomfortable around people, or you may have learned a defense mechanism—that conscious mental process built-in to protect you. To protect your ego, you decide you want to avoid criticism, internal anxiety, or ostracism and thereby remain as "unseen" as possible. I can relate to this for sure!

No matter the psychological type you start to pattern, all human behaviors are shaped (some might say predetermined) by the size of the family you come from, the positive or negative people around you, the levels of nurturance you receive, and the groups that you attach yourself to as you mature. You start discovering some of the nature-given strengths you were born with, whether good looks, a sense of humor, a strong athletic ability, or high intelligence, and you start to define who you want to become.

But be forewarned; these gifts don't come free. Where one strength rules, there are many weaknesses just waiting to oppose. The conscious and subconscious are in constant struggle.

You start to juggle life and realize you need to decide what you are going to do with it. Perhaps go to college or become a top athlete, and in this dreaming, wishing, hoping, and working toward some goals or aspirations, you start to experience new thoughts and understandings. For example, "This is much harder than I thought it would be. What was I thinking?" However, with persistence and a few successes under your belt, you become cognizant of the fact that you might actually have a talent and might even be the master of your own destiny!

You start to know who you are. You start to define and determine who you are. It feels great. You are in charge!

Or, so you think.

Because just as you think you have that mastered, something steps in the way. Or as John Lennon sang, "Life is (just) what happens to you while you are busy making other plans."

LIFE CONTINUALLY EVOLVES

With these few successes, and hopefully many more failures behind you, your life evolves. And for most people, we become less egocentric and start to crave deeper relationships and bonds. This has its good and bad sides because it encourages you to create new relationships, but as time goes on you find yourself, sadly, losing those you love either because of different belief systems, or worse yet, illness and death. I know, I've had that pain and it has changed my life.

No matter how much you think you are in control, your deeper underlying purpose and virtue and the cycle of life can't be ignored. You carry memories within you of all sorts, and you get molded and defined by each action and reaction. That is science. That is nature. That is faith and spirituality.

But you persevere again, and now it is your turn to start to teach others what you have learned yourself. You may start to have children of your own, or you may go into teaching or instructing, or a life of service, or you may decide that no, you want none of that because you are on the top of your game and this is the time for you to shine. It is the constant roller coaster of growing pains of life and love and the dichotomies I refer to as the "karmic cul-de-sac"; disappointment and fulfillment; challenges and opportunities; failure and success... and failure, again, and the next thing you know you are a professional, in your mid-fifties, just like me, and it feels as though life has just flown by. Of the many life lessons I've learned over the years, there is a need for failure, and in some cases massive failure! Because, ultimately, it's the experience of failure that provides us the momentum to swing in the other direction toward success. Never fear failure; instead, embrace it, and use it as a wake-up call to move toward huge success.

A weird convergence transpires: The lines or roads and crazy detours seem to make uncanny sense because they have led you to this exact moment. Well, that moment for me is what this book, The PRISE Life, is all about.

As a scientist, I have carefully analyzed, written, studied, restudied, taught, and looked at data from all angles. I have spent my life trying to figure out why we humans react and act as we do. In my case, my passion has been through human nutrition and applied physiology. And although it started as a more egocentric need to be the best athlete I could, and to beat all others in competition whether it was hockey, tennis, triathlons, etc., there was an internal drive in me pushing to be the best.

I never really thought about it in this way until I started giving speeches. Now I know this convergence was probably no accident at all.

The daily lessons of failure, trial and error, and rough times all converged. Whatever life had in mind, it eventually created the momentum I needed to develop resolve and a healthy dose of spiritual and emotional fulfillment combined with nutrition and smart/safe levels of exercise.

I have learned that development, then balance, also applies to nutrition, and is something I have researched more. The life cycle of plants I learned in the garden with my mother so many years ago is just as crucial as the psychological life cycle of humans and has so many things to teach us.

LESSONS FROM MOTHER EARTH

Mother Earth is, undoubtedly, still the prime nourisher, and if we focus on the quality of soil, replenishing enzymes, and restoring agriculture, as it was supposed to be without all the added chemicals and pesticides, and replace what minerals have been robbed from us while focusing on high-quality (whole) foods and even supplements, we will become a healthier world. The garden teaches us everything we need to know in life: When to plant a seed, when and how much water is needed, getting necessary sunshine and when it's time to be in the shade, how to grow strong or rest, when to add extra nourishment when some quality is missing, when to remove bugs and when to add bugs.

The whole cycle of human nutrition can be found in the seasons, in gardening, and in the organisms. It is an environment that supports all life. Nurturing a living organism through its life cycle is physically and spiritually one of the most significant actions one can participate in. It's something I encourage everyone to try because there are deeply satisfying feelings when you bring food fresh from your garden right to your table. You will find it bursting with so much flavor that you will probably wonder why you didn't try it sooner.

Eating foods that contain all the vital and essential nutrients (vitamins, minerals, phytochemicals) that originate primarily from the earth or garden, or even today in reputable nature-based supplements and meal-replacement protein powders and bars, make us strong. This is the epitome of the modern-day, plant-based lifestyle and one that I fully support. Fake foods, which often lead to unhealthy cravings and addictions, make us weak. But by combining healthy nutrition with exercise and fitness routines, research has proven that a smart integration will net significant mood-enhancement. We all feel better, have more energy, and think more clearly when we fuel our bodies with nutritious, healthy food.

You hear about the "runner's high" and have probably experienced that exuberance after a really challenging, but fun, team sport, being active outdoors in nature, or a time you pushed yourself further than ever before. All these actions create endorphins, as well as other positive biochemical reactions, and in combination help your body support your mind. Positive thinking is so much easier when you feel good, right?

THE SCIENCE MATTERS

The stages of my life, with the types of emotional, physical, spiritual, "nutrition," and at times "deprivation," as well as quantifiable research, have been invaluable as I have tried to make sense of achieving optimal health and peak performance. I moved from that egocentric world of wanting to figure out how to be the best athlete I could be, to discovering that I liked helping others even more. This gave me a deeper sense of fulfillment and meaning.

This is what drives me today. To inspire others to embrace their health and take control of their daily lifestyle choices is what has pushed me to work so hard and want to take a risk, not only to write this book but share the gifts that have been given to me. The need to show others how to improve their overall health and fitness, with scientific proof to back it up, has consumed me, but it now makes sense. The result: My brainchild (the program that has become popularly referred to as Dr. Paul's PRISE Life Protocol, this overarching lifestyle program) was born. The execution of daily lifestyle strategies that bring the most health benefit to all individuals no matter their shape, size, health, diet, or experience level.

In other words, PRISE is a comprehensive, holistic and integrative lifestyle of nutrition, fitness and mind/brain health strategies. How to actually feed the body with life-giving nutrients, movement and mindfulness are what keeps me coming back. The success stories I hear daily, the response from audiences, the thrill of changing lives for the better, that is a blessed life.

My overall goal with this book, and in the coming years, is to continue to educate people, provide resources, give speeches—to as many as will listen—through live audiences and now through the incredible world of the internet and web, social media, print, etc.so that others can learn that there is an easier way to maintain and attain optimal health and peak performance. I want people to hear it from a real scientist, not an "expert" who happened upon something that worked for them alone, not from a "celebrity" who already has a predefined audience, but from a true scientist who through years of research, statistics, experiments, human studies, and relationships truly happened upon such amazing results that I can no longer keep them to myself!

The bottom line is, we all know of people who struggle with ill health or can't make that leap to exercise or lose weight, and because they have gone about it the wrong way in the past they have given up. No more!

WHAT TO EXPECT IN THIS BOOK

I have purposefully written this book in an easy-to-read manner and taken my scientist lab coat off to make sure that the studies are easily understood. The value of the research results and recommendations can be executed immediately in your own life. However, should the scientist in you need to read through the scientific studies and data to find your own validations, all the details of research and studies can be found on my website: www.priselife.com.

By the end of this book, you will understand The PRISE Life, and, pardon the pun, you will have won the prize. With that magic something I call Protein Pacing, you will finally have the chance to be the best you can be. You will learn what is entailed in scientific research with terms such as third-party independent research, original investigations, right of first refusal, full disclosure, peer-reviewed, and other facts that will help you become a discriminating reader and chooser of the type of lifestyle you determine you would like to live. Not a diet. A truly healthy and everlasting lifestyle. And, as I play on Hamlet's words from his famous soliloquy, you do have the right "To be or not to be"… healthy. (See, I did learn something from high school after all.)

Most importantly, I want you to choose health. Not just survive, but have true optimal health. La dolce vita, as they say in Italian. The sweet life.

YOUR FIRST ACTION STEP

Right now, please download The PRISE Life app. It's free! And enter your details so you can follow along with a PRISE Life plan that best suits your age, weight, gender and desired level of activity. I will guide you with video tutorials and we can connect on my Facebook page, 'PRISE Life,' and my website.

Please, have patience with yourself. Find enjoyment and mental strength along the way. That is why I am here to show you the way, the pace, for the ultimate race: a healthy and vibrant life.

Finally, remember, the human body is a complicated but perfectly designed mechanism, and we are still in the early stages of understanding everything about it. Embrace it. Embrace your body and type, even as it is today. Embrace your God-given virtue most of all. Embrace the stages and ages of your life. They go by more quickly than you think. Don't lose them to bad information, ill health, and negative emotions. Heed the information, follow the steps and take it one day at a time, because with those few pieces in order you will achieve more than you ever imagined. Take it from a half-a-centurion: Don't miss one moment along the way, even if life is making other plans for you. One day it will all make sense. And always, always stay positive and "Keep your eyes on the PRISE!"

CHAPTER 2
THE STORY BEHIND PRISE®

Never get so busy making a living
that you forget to make a life.
— Aristotle

Who knew my early start with The PRISE Life actually began when I was competing as an athlete eager for new ways to enhance my performance and recovery from training and competitions? It exploded when others started looking to me for advice, but the next journey I am going to share ends with a very different moral to the story than you may guess, so please read to the very end.

THE ACCIDENTAL EXPERT

In my peak years of athletic competition, I began doing all sorts of nutrition, physiology, and scientific-based research to help me improve. But, over time, more and more people started asking me what I was doing to stay in shape and perform at a high level. The sharing of this information with others actually became more fulfilling and motivating to me. But I knew I had "arrived" when my own research was being accepted in peer-reviewed publications and leading science journals, and I was sought as an invited speaker at various national and international nutrition and sports medicine conferences.

I was quickly becoming one of the go-to content experts in my field. It seemed everyone was looking to get healthy and fit. As a matter of fact, when I would send out announcements in local newspapers looking for interested study participants to learn more about enrolling in one of my upcoming research studies, I was blown away by the number of people who would show up in my small community just for the informational meetings—sometimes as many as 240 people! This is unheard of in terms of human clinical intervention studies that involve a nutrition and exercise program. I knew I was onto something special.

I've often been asked how I came up with The PRISE Protocol, which stands for P-Protein Pacing, R- Resistance, I- Intervals, S- Stretching and E- Endurance. We'll talk more about these individual components in the following chapter. We'll talk about why they work in the second half of the book. It might surprise you, but the reason I developed PRISE is that current exercise and nutrition recommendations are too time-consuming, confusing, and unrealistic for most people.

SIMPLE STATISTICS WITH BIG RESULTS

The truth is that less than 20% of the United States population follows a healthy, active lifestyle program on a consistent basis, but in the research studies I have conducted using The PRISE Life Protocol, the participant compliance is often 80% or higher! That's astronomical! People love The PRISE Life because it's easy to follow and consistently produces results. People report their excitement because they don't feel like they are being held hostage to a diet and exercise plan, but feel as though they can actually incorporate this as a lifestyle change for the rest of their lives. Now that's proof of its success!

I developed PRISE in response to the exercise and nutrition recommendations from the leading organizations in the world, including the American College of Sports Medicine (ACSM), the American Heart Association (AHA), The Obesity Society (TOS), and the Institute of Medicine (IOM). But while the current exercise recommendations are very well-intentioned and well-meaning, they are not feasible for the vast majority of the population to achieve.

Being a Fellow in the ACSM since 1997 and having served on the AHA advisory board, as well as being a Fellow in the TOS and the International Society of Sports Nutrition (ISSN), my aim is not to criticize these leading organizations of health and wellness. They are doing great work. The statistics I cite are meant to steer us in a new direction. They are a guidepost to address a glaring disconnect I have witnessed over the past few decades. Most importantly, my research, which is cited favorably in many of these well-respected journals and reviewed by my peers, means I truly am a leading scientist. The best feeling to me is that I am contributing to the current exercise and nutrition recommendations, which are helping pave the way for more people to regain and maintain their health.

BACK TO THE BASICS

Let's go back to the basics and look at what actually being recommended. I calculated the number of hours necessary to accomplish the current recommendations, and can you believe that it requires up to fourteen hours a week! That is equivalent to two hours per day of exercise!

The truth is, most people are busy. Very few people have time to exercise every day. Ninety minutes a day (especially for those who are not exercising at all) is too overwhelming and unrealistic. Not only are the current recommendations too extreme and time-consuming, but they are also confusing to follow and, most importantly, make no connection to healthy eating. Thus, I wanted to develop a more sensible exercise routine that embraced all the important components of the current requirements but was also seamlessly connected to a simple nutrition lifestyle strategy. This is how PRISE was born.

The very strange thing about life is that we often don't know what is motivating us while we are deep in it, and it's not until we are forced to slow down or asked to summarize our lives that all of a sudden we get new perspectives. Someone recently shared this quote by Aristotle with me: "Never get so busy making a living that you forget to make a life." The timing was perfect. I'm so grateful for the little signs that pop up along the way to show we are on the right track.

THE EPIPHANY OF PRISE

While writing this book, I was strongly encouraged to think further about how I pioneered Protein Pacing along with The PRISE Life Protocol. In a moment of clarity, it was like the blinders had been taken off of me. All along I thought that I was looking for the best way an athlete could reach their peak performance, but I realized The PRISE Life was so much more than that. The fact is, I created this protocol out of survival.

"Why survival?" you might be asking. Early in my professorial career as a scientist, when my wife, Karen, and I had our first two sons, ages one and three at the time, we both had full-time jobs and were juggling. We were trying to nurture our marriage, navigate our still new roles as parents, deal with regular life stress, balance new careers, pay the bills, and well, just trying to survive. Maybe you've been there too? I call it, "Struggle of the Juggle." All of that with absolutely no downtime.

NO BREAKS FOR A BUSY SCIENTIST

Let me give you just a little background. After graduating with two master's degrees, a doctorate, and having done postdoctoral fellowship training, I was fortunate enough to get a full-time faculty position at a prestigious four-year liberal arts college as an untenured professor, and on top of that, I was the head men's tennis coach. As a college professor and scientific scholar with a lab, I was the two-for-the-price-of-one guy. Yup, my total salary of $32,000 a year, for a family of four, came with two jobs—and may I say, two jobs that had completely opposing schedules. Meanwhile, Karen was working as a physical therapist and was an amazing mom to our two beautiful babies.

Leave it to me to choose a more difficult route than I thought I was taking. Other scientists joke that they have more flexibility working with a mouse or a cell because they can do it on their time. Working with the human metabolism meant starting at 5–6:00 a.m. on every laboratory testing day, taking samples and working with my subjects. Starting so early meant leaving my wife to care for the babies. I would run to the lab, get my tests done, run back home to help feed the babies breakfast, then take over so my wife could get to work.

Fortunately, the boys' daycare was in the building next to my office, so I would drop them off and head in to teach classes, grade papers and exams, do research, serve on committees, write manuscripts for publication, apply for grant and research funding, and by about 4:00 p.m. when others at the college were clearing out and going home to be with their families and rest up, where was I headed? Well, to my job as head tennis coach, of course! It started at about 4:00 p.m., when the athletes would show up and practice, and depending on the season could go on until after 7:00 p.m.

There were even days during the late winter and early spring that I started before 5:00 a.m. and got off after midnight because the courts were booked and we'd have to start practice at 10:00 p.m. But that's not all. I was also the team driver! On many Friday nights, my wife was dropping off cookies and cakes for our team, with two kids on her arms, so I could drive up to six hours to the next competition.

I was often gone all Friday night, all Saturday, and late into Sunday, and would only get home in time to grade papers, plan my lessons, do my research, write up information and keep the committees happy. I was even in charge of recruiting. Your head is spinning in circles, to be honest, and the more my wife and I discussed this, the more we couldn't believe we did it for twelve years! Mostly, we did it because we considered my players and students our adopted children; we loved them and would do anything for them. But life was stressful for sure.

When you're in it you just do what you need to do, and we were definitely living at max velocity! We still wonder how it took us so long to wake up and realize how much we sacrificed ourselves along the way. It's probably because we were stuck in survival mode and never took a breath to contemplate what we were really doing and what the consequences were. We needed to figure out how to get out of the rat race, or at least slow down the wheel! I'm sharing this because there is a very real possibility in today's world that you are in the same spot we were.

THE PRACTICALITY OF PRISE

Maybe you can imagine spending so little time with your children and your husband or wife. Maybe you too are stuck spending hours working around the clock? Maybe, like me, you have no assistant at work; and no extra help. Or maybe you have been struggling with your health and fitness your entire life and don't know who to believe or where to turn for help. I understand life can be really brutal at times.

Now, imagine running that much on so little. What does that do to a person? Maybe you can guess because you are living this way too? It's exhausting. Finding time to nurture yourself to be the best parent, spouse and professional you can be is not easy.

Because I was a scientist in health and nutrition I knew I had to keep up and remain emotionally balanced and fit. But how? I created my own plan! Yes, one that was effective and healthy and didn't take as much time as my profession told me it should. Out of my own necessity, I created a nutrition and exercise plan for people who have no time or simply don't know what to do. Can you believe I only realized this recently?

I needed to incorporate the healthiest and quickest eating and staying-healthy program I could find. I was not going to sacrifice my love for my family. I had to figure out how to get some exercise in, how I could maintain my muscle strength and function, and how I could perform my job and also be a devoted husband and father without getting fatigued. I simply couldn't risk letting anyone down or letting my job duties slip because I was too tired, ill, or hurt.

Additionally, I had to figure out how to properly stretch in limited times, and how to keep my heart functioning at peak levels to build endurance because I was literally on the run for my life! This was the most absurd, chaotic, and crazy life I could imagine, and I was trying everything in my power to stay alive and healthy while achieving my goals and maintaining my responsibilities to my career and family. Throughout all of this, my top priority was staying close to my family. When this was challenged, I went into high-alert mode. It is often reported that the greatest contributions are born out of survival and the protection of loved ones. In my case, PRISE was due to both.

A WELCOME CHANGE

It was a full twelve years before the college came to me and gave me a choice. Ironically, they, not me, realized that my two full-time jobs were pretty close to humanly impossible. I was given the choice to either be a scientist or the head tennis coach. And as you can probably guess, I chose scientist. But the coach in me has never diminished and is one of the main reasons I decided to write this book.

I am grateful to the administration for realizing that what I was doing was nearly impossible, and perhaps because they were looking from the outside in, they could see those circles I was running in that I couldn't see myself. Are you doing the same thing? Are you running in circles or finding it so hard to keep up that you can't see what or why you are doing it? Is there a better way? Can that way start now?

I don't want you to live through what we did. I want you to learn from our mistakes, and that means, first, stop, take a breath, and ask yourself, "Is everything I'm doing really necessary?" I want you to ask yourself that question seriously. Why? Because one of the largest research groups I ended up studying included working moms juggling life, career, kids, family, money, health, finances, love, stress, and the list goes on. I would look at their commitment (and the busy men as well) and realize that so many of the people who strive to do well, watch what they eat, and try to get in exercise are overachievers just like me.

WELCOME TO THE PRISE LIFE TEAM

To become part of The PRISE Life team you only have to do a few things and we will all be winners together.

Download The PRISE Life app and program in your protocol.

Join me on Facebook on our PRISE Life page. I go LIVE frequently and I'd love to meet you there. Be sure to drop a thumbs up or comment and say hello.

Tag us on Instagram @drpaularciero and @priselife. Show us how you're moving and eating well and we'll cheer you on every step of the way.

We need you to be a part of this PRISE Life team. We want you to say yes to a healthier way of life that is scientifically proven to support your vitality and longevity. From the very core of who I am, I want to help YOU. Let's reassess what you are doing and allow me to teach you how to make nutrition and fitness an easier, more permanent, part of your life.

Ask yourself, "What can I let go of to enhance the quality of my life, and who can help me?" The beauty of my life's lesson, which was completely out of balance back then, was that I had the desperation to create The PRISE Life Protocol that will help put your life back into balance too. I encourage you to fully embrace this program. With millions of others as living proof, you too can achieve optimal health and peak performance with a busy schedule.

If we had a chance to do things over, I would never have gotten so busy making a living that I lost, forever, the time to make a life. Fortunately, as my PRISE LIfe Protocol became more and more refined, I was able to spend more and more time with Karen and my kids. They were, and always will remain, my PRISE. Please, please do not make the same mistakes I did. Together we are all going to hold each other accountable to work smarter and not harder! Do you promise? I do. I'm committed to making life better for all of us.

Amazingly, through these three decades, one of the most astonishing results of my research still stands: What we are being taught and told to do in the area of nutrition and exercise has missed the target and may be causing more harm to our bodies than healing and strengthening us.

Every time I share my work and see results, I feel more driven to share this with the world. I have made this protocol simple and easy to follow.

Over these next five chapters, I'm excited to show you exactly how The PRISE Life works and how to incorporate each of these lifestyle strategies into your daily life, so you can reach optimal health and peak performance. It is easier than you might think! If I and countless others can do it, then you can, too!

Together, we can stop obesity, improve poor health, and teach the world that you don't have to fall for the misinformation that is out there. Have the courage to put your belief in this. You really can, and will, achieve success by following The PRISE Life. You will find that this protocol is the answer to Aristotle's sage advice: "Never get so busy making a living that you forget to make a life."

CHAPTER 3

(P) IS FOR PROTEIN PACING

Adopt the pace of nature: Her secret is patience.
— Ralph Waldo Emerson

PROTEIN PACING | RESISTANCE | INTERVAL | STRETCHING | ENDURANCE

You may say, "I have tried every diet or lifestyle change out there, Dr. Paul. Why will this one work?" It's a big thing you might never have heard of called Protein Pacing. It all comes down to this one major revelation. There is one common denominator among all of these various diets that all nutrition and diet experts agree on, and I am the nutrition scientist who developed this nutritional strategy. Let's get started!

From a dietary intake standpoint, human survival has always required a critical amount of protein intake because so many life-sustaining functions and structures depend on protein consumption. Our early ancestors ate what they hunted and often consumed foods that were also high in fat to sustain them through times of famine. We then supported our quick energy needs with plants, especially nuts and seeds. This is what made us strong enough to go out and tend to the land or hunt for dinner or pick those vegetables and berries from the wild. Mother Nature has taught and continues to teach us everything we need to know. We simply need to start listening.

WHAT'S THE BIG DEAL WITH PROTEIN PACING?

We have probably all heard the Hypocrites quote: "Let food be thy medicine." I would add, "Pick the right ones and then time them properly." What many consider to be my most important scientific discovery was the observation that by consuming ideal amounts of high-quality protein (20–40 grams per serving) four to six times per day (with and without exercise training), people reduced total body and abdominal fat to a greater extent than the typically consumed three traditional higher-carbohydrate meals per day. This work was published in the *Obesity Journal* in 2013 (Impact Factor: 4.3) and the *Journal of Applied Physiology* in 2014 (Impact Factor: 3.4) and led to the terms "Protein Pacing" and "PRISE Life Protocol," as well as numerous additional peer-reviewed publications.

In fact, the highly acclaimed monthly medical newsletter Duke Medicine Health News published a four-page feature article highlighting my PRISE Life Protocol and Protein Pacing research. In addition, my research has been extensively cited in other medical publications such as the AHA (American Heart Association), Science Daily and Villanova COPE.

My PRISE Life protocol has also been cited in mainstream popular media, including *The Wall Street Journal, Fox News, Prevention, Good Housekeeping, WebMD, O Magazine, TIME, Huffington Post, Daily Mail, SELF, Glamour, Shape, Health, Women's Health, Women's World, Muscle and Fitness, Men's Fitness, and Men's Health*. Other national media outlets include *Doctor Radio XM/Sirius, Guru Performance, and Rusty Lion Podcast* on iTunes. The National Public Radio program *Academic Minute, Best of Our Knowledge* has not only featured my research but also awarded me with the 2015 Most Likely to Change the World Senior Superlative Award. I'm also a member of the International Protein Board, comprised of the top protein scientists in the world (www.internationalproteinboard.org).

With all that shared, I don't need to tell you that most weight-loss plans don't work over the long term. You inherently know this. That's why I wanted to share all the research and recognition The PRISE Life has drawn in over the years, so you can feel completely optimistic about Protein Pacing. This will be the routine that changes your body—and your life—for good.

THE COURAGE TO BEGIN AGAIN

Success is never final, failure is never fatal.
It's courage that counts.
— John Wooden

Courage! Depending on where you are at with food, nutrition, and exercise, The PRISE Life will either become the simple fix that is missing from your current diet or your awakening to see that the answers are here and that you can absolutely make these easy changes in your daily routine for dramatic success. No matter what your situation is, this will help you create a permanent and sustainable lifestyle of healthy eating and reasonable exercise. As I also said in the beginning, there is no downside to this protocol, and if you follow it as I have set it up, there is guaranteed scientific success. Few, if any, other doctors or experts to date can say that!

The fact is that people are still confused about what they should be eating and how they should be exercising. How do I know? Because thousands upon thousands of books have been written on the subject and people are still obese and confused and sick. And because other experts are seeking me out for advice, millions upon millions are now looking at my research and quoting or following it.

Believe me when I assure you that this program is different. From the get-go, my primary research goal has been about improving health through changing a person's body composition, reducing fat, and increasing muscle tone so they're performing at peak condition. I just knew there was a way to get the body to burn more fuel, specifically fat fuel, by optimizing what, when, and how a person eats and what type of exercise they do.

It took a few decades (and dozens of extensive scientific studies, beginning in 1988) to home in on the ideal formulation, but several years ago I finally devised the perfect nutrition plan, one that I wrote up for the March 2013 edition of the highly regarded scientific journal Obesity, and have since reproduced in several groundbreaking, published studies.

MASSIVE RESULTS

In the first-of-its-kind study, I detailed how men and women who followed a reasonable, deprivation-free Protein Pacing diet plan, without any exercise, were able to shed up to 5.5 pounds in one week and eleven pounds in four weeks. This weight wasn't just water loss. I calculated fat loss, too, and some dieters shed 12.5 pounds of body fat, including 2.5 pounds of belly fat, all while building lean body (muscle) mass (up to four pounds!) after just eight weeks!

That means belts tightened, dress sizes dropped, and body changes felt and seen. In a recent follow-up study, I tested my Protein Pacing plan in a group of forty overweight men and women, and in twelve weeks they lost an average of 10% body weight or twenty-four pounds, with some losing up to sixty-five pounds, nine inches off their waist circumference, and forty-six pounds of fat, including more than four pounds of belly fat!

Remarkably, despite the massive loss of body weight and body fat, the relative amount of healthy lean muscle mass increased by 9%! In seven follow-up studies, I added exercise to the Protein Pacing equation (using my PRISE Life protocol details I am sharing with you in the next part) and the results were off the charts—by adding four short workouts a week to this program, you could lose as much as twenty-two pounds in four weeks! And these results are not just for those interested in weight loss.

I've tested my PRISE Life Protocol on super-fit men and women, and they too outperformed their non-PRISE counterparts in every measure of physical performance! Imagine finally knowing that you can end the diet roller coaster and enjoy a program that keeps you healthy but does not deprive you.

THE RULES OF PROTEIN PACING

The rules of the Protein Pacing eating plan came from years of performing my own research and from reading scientific studies from my colleagues. I pulled the best parts from each of these plans, meshed them together with some of my own work, and landed on an eating routine that produced the best results I've ever encountered. And it holds true to this day!

So just what is this magical lifestyle formula? Well, it's not nearly as complicated as you might think. In fact, it borrows from principles that you may have seen before. Here are the basics of the Protein Pacing plan:

Each Protein Pacing snack or meal should include a high-quality complete protein of all twenty amino acids from either animal or plant-based or a combination of both.

- Each snack or meal should contain 20–40g of high-quality protein.
- Eat four to six Protein Pacing snacks or meals per day.
- Evenly space your meals (about every three to four hours) throughout the day.

- Eat your first Protein Pacing meal sixty minutes from waking in the morning. This is what I refer to as the Morning Muscle Maximizer (MMM).
- Eat your last meal within two hours of going to sleep at night. This is what I call the Bedtime Belly fat Burner (BBB).

When it comes to eating, quality and moderation—not deprivation—are the keys to controlling cravings and sticking with a healthy lifestyle. If you want to lose weight, place the right amount and type of protein (20-40g) and fats (saturated, monounsaturated) on your plate and less simple and refined carbohydrates.

Four to six meals a day keeps your metabolism roaring and decreases your chance of unplanned snacking, as long as you are eating protein at each of these meals! Eating the right carbohydrates keeps your blood sugar and insulin at healthy levels. Fueling your body with the right fat can help decrease inflammation in your blood vessels, enhance brain and nerve function, and provide an excellent energy source for physical activity. Natural whole and nutrient-dense engineered foods—not heavily engineered nutrient-deficient ones—are best because they contain the ideal amount and ratio of cancer-fighting phytonutrients, vitamins, and minerals necessary to help us prevent disease and perform at our best. By eating foods that are more filling, you won't miss any extra calories you give up.

Download The PRISE Life app now to get a personalized plan just for you. When I tested hundreds of people on The PRISE Life Protocol, they experienced weight loss so significant that I was sure they were hungry or deprived or tired, which are common side effects of consuming too little fuel. They weren't! Instead, these men and women lost fat, flab, jiggle, and belly rolls, all while feeling better than ever. And you can too! The Protein Pacing plan is designed to help you burn more fat calories all day and build more lean muscle, all while keeping you feeling satisfied and not hungry. Many reported experiencing a happier, less-stressed mood state as well on the Protein Pacing meal plan.

The beauty of Protein Pacing is that it can fit into anyone's busy lifestyle and food preferences, intolerances, and allergies. Below, I show you how easy it is to include my Protein Pacing plan into any nutrition/diet plan you choose. For example, the growing popularity of the plant-based, Mediterranean, Paleolithic, and fat-adapted/ketogenic diets meet the needs of those of you wanting to kick start your weight loss or enjoy an athletic performance advantage over your competition.

Here are some sample meal plan breakdowns:

The Optimal Protein Pacing plan:	The Protein Pacing Mediterranean plan:
30% protein 30% fat 40% carbs	20%–25% protein 25%–30% fat 50% carbs
The Protein Pacing Plant-based plan:	The Protein Pacing Paleolithic plan:
20%–25% protein 15%–20% fats 60%–70% carbs	20%–30% protein 50%–60% fat 20%–40% carbs
The Protein Pacing fat-adapted/ketogenic plan:	
20% protein 70%–75% fat 10%–15% carbs	

Regardless of the nutrition plan you choose, Protein Pacing is always the foundational core. This is why I'm so passionate about spreading the word on Protein Pacing. It is the common nutrition thread to EVERY nutrition/diet plan available!

A PROTEIN PACING PRIMER

Our bodies thrive on a diet consisting of 25%-35% lean, healthy protein (from both plant and animal sources; roughly 20–40g of protein per meal), along with at least 25% healthy fats and oils and lots of fresh veggies, certain whole grains, and fruits. Performing a combination of exercise routines, as opposed to just one or two different types, on a weekly basis results in drastic health and physical-performance improvements.

Protein Pacing holds the key to weight loss. I believe we need to be more inclusive (not divisive) and promote a balanced nutritional eating landscape that doesn't alienate one food group from another. A balance of high-quality, nutrient-dense whole foods from local and/or organic plant and animal sources are best for optimal health. Both animal and plant-based diets provide superior health benefits. We just need to focus on the quality of the source of each and find more harmony in our nutritional recommendations.

Like almost anything consumable, not all available foods are created equal. While it is true that good food can be expensive, it is best to always minimize the toxins in your food while maximizing nutrition and health benefits from every item that enters your body (I discuss this in more detail in Chapter 9). The most obvious argument in favor of more expensive food is that healthier people spend less money on health care in the future! Healthy, organic, local, humanely raised, small farm produce, meat, and dairy take more work to produce and are thus more expensive. But this food is also better for you, it tastes better, and its purchase gives money back to your local communities.

Not everyone has access to these resources but, whenever you can, endeavor to buy (in order of importance): unprocessed/raw/pure (no additives, just the thing you want!), organic (non-GMO and without chemicals or synthetic pesticides), and local food. If you must prioritize which foods to spend more money on, choose lots of plants (vegetables, nuts, seeds, legumes, whole grains, fruits), fish, meat, dairy, and eggs. In general, foods containing more fat store far more toxins than non-fatty foods do, making their quality of utmost importance. For example, scientific evidence has shown that grass-fed animal sources (beef, dairy, eggs, etc.) have higher nutritional content and a much healthier fatty acid profile than factory-farmed animal sources, especially beef, dairy and poultry And the same goes for organic produce.

When you go to the grocery store, take this book so you can reference these important lists as you shop. These are many of the foods that are a staple in my diet and on the Protein Pacing plan.

PROTEIN PACING IN ACTION:

On this plan, I recommend eating 20–40g of protein per sitting. This is the amount that will keep you feeling full and properly fueled until your next mini-meal in a few hours.

Plant-based Proteins

- Legumes (beans): adzuki, black, cannellini, garbanzo, navy, kidney, pinto, soy beans, edamame (eat 8–12 oz.)
- Peas: split peas, lentils, black-eyed peas (eat 8–12 oz.)
- Moringa (3 oz.)
- Tofu, tempeh, and seitan (eat 5–7 oz.)
- Nuts: macadamia, pistachio, walnut, almond, pecan, peanut, cashew (eat 3.5 oz. unsalted, raw or dry-roasted). Some nuts, such as cashews and peanuts, can also be significant sources of carbohydrates.
- Seeds: raw pumpkin (pepitas), sunflower, flax, chia (3.5 oz. unsalted or salted)

Animal Proteins

(Please refer to my cookbook for a more detailed list)

- Fish: haddock, cod, scrod, halibut, catfish, crawfish, flounder, herring, perch, sole, trout, clam, tuna, salmon, mackerel, sardines, anchovies, snapper, mahi-mahi, shellfish (eat 3.5 oz.)
- Eggs: cooked egg whites (eat four egg whites), hardboiled (eat three eggs), scrambled (eat three eggs), egg substitute (eat 5–7 oz.)
- Yogurt: Greek yogurt, plain, unsweetened (eat 8 oz.); Greek yogurt, plain, 2% (eat 8.5 oz.); kefir, plain, low-fat (eat 14 oz.); regular yogurt, non/low-fat, plain: (eat 16 oz.)
- Cottage cheese: Nonfat cottage cheese (eat 5.5 oz.), 1% low-fat cottage cheese (eat 6 oz.), 2% cottage cheese (eat 8 oz.), 4% cottage cheese (eat 7 oz.)
- Milk: whole, preferably from grass-fed cows (drink 20 oz.)
- Meat: grass-fed beef, sirloin, or buffalo (eat 3.5 oz.); organic chicken breast (eat 2.5 oz.); chicken, dark meat (eat 2.5 oz.); sliced turkey or ham, try to avoid cold cuts high in sodium or with added sugars (eat 3.5 oz.); ground turkey (eat 3 oz.); turkey breast (2.5 oz.); turkey dark meat (2.5 oz.); pork chop (eat 3 oz.); pork tenderloin (eat 3 oz.).

Don't forget to add your supplements:

- Whey protein
- Pea protein
- Legume (fava, mung, bean) protein, brown rice protein
- Hemp protein
- Bone broth protein
- Collagen protein
- Moringa protein

Get Your Fats:

- Saturated: Grass-fed butter and clarified butter (ghee); grass-fed beef tallow; duck fat; full-fat yogurt
- Monounsaturated: Cold-pressed organic extra virgin olive oil (EVOO), avocados, macadamia nuts, almonds, cashews, pistachios
- Polyunsaturated: Omega-6s and omega-3s from krill oil/sardines, wild-caught salmon; small fish, not farmed, not grain or factory food fed
- Get Your Carbs: To maximize nutrient intake per calorie and minimize empty carbs that are easily transformed into glucose (fat forming at high levels), the majority of your carbohydrates should come in the form of fresh vegetables, resistant starches that I described earlier, and some high-nutrient fruits and berries.
- Portion: Eat vegetables with three or more of your four to six daily mini-meals. Green leafy vegetables can be eaten in abundance, but steam them once they exceed a fist-sized portion.
- Grains in Moderation: Quinoa, barley, steel-cut oats, wild/brown rice, spelt, resistant starches (refer to my discussion of "Wonder Carbs" in Chapter 11 and my cookbook to help guide you through your choices).
- Vegetables: Broccoli, kale, escarole, chicory, swiss chard, spinach, collard greens, beet greens, masculine (can often be a greens salad mix), summer and fall squashes (pumpkin, acorn, butternut), beets, carrots, tomatoes, avocado.
- Fruits in moderation: Pomegranate, bananas, melons, peaches, mango, oranges, grapefruit, pineapple, kiwi, apples, pears, nectarines, plums
- Berries: Blueberries, blackberries, acai berries, raspberries, boysenberries, strawberries, cranberries

GRAB-AND-GO OPTIONS

If you want to start working your way toward this Protein Pacing style of eating right now—before you even make a trip to the store—I've made this list of fifteen snack and mini-meal options that can be eaten right out of your crisper or pantry. These are good grab-and-go options for travel or during the workday. I make sure I have plenty of these ingredients on hand at all times so I can satisfy any cravings that strike, be it for salty foods or sweet ones.

15 Protein Pacing snacks you can eat right now:

- A banana and a handful of almonds.
- A couple of hard-boiled eggs.
- A cup of full fat cottage cheese with avocado, sprouts, some nuts or blueberries.
- A glass or two of 10 grams of protein unsweetened almond, hemp, or coconut milk with high-fiber whole-grain crackers, veggies and nut butter.
- A cup of unsweetened full-fat Greek yogurt (preferably from entirely grass-fed cows) with fresh fruit.
- Whole grain rice cakes with nut or seed butter and sliced fruit with a glass of milk (dairy, almond, coconut, cashew). Remember that dairy milk has roughly 12g of lactose (milk sugar) per cup. Other milks may prove just as satisfying without the empty carbohydrates.
- Homemade hummus with veggies.
- Mixed greens and a can of tuna in water. (If you can find it, tuna in extra virgin olive oil is also a delicious quick meal. Beware of inflammatory vegetable oils, such as canola and soybean oil).
- Pita wrap with chicken, turkey, or fish and fresh veggies.
- A berry smoothie with a scoop of a pea, brown rice, fava, mung, hemp, moringa, or undenatured whey protein.

- Apple slices with natural (preferably organic) nut or seed butter (again, look out for added vegetable oils, particularly hydrogenated oils, which are used to extend shelf life and maintain a thick consistency).
- A handful of assorted nuts and dried fruit (do your best to avoid dried fruit with added sugar. If you let your taste buds adjust, you will find that unsweetened dried fruit is packed with condensed fruit sugars).
- 1 cup of canned or cooked beans (lentils, black/kidney beans, chickpeas, etc.) with rice or quinoa.
- Homemade turkey meatball pita wrap.
- 10 oz. of (unsweetened or lightly sweetened, grass-fed) kefir with almonds or walnuts.
- Protein powders, bars or snacks (homemade or store-bought—see my approved list of bars).

PROTEIN PACING TIMING CHART

The chart provided here shows a simple schedule for meal timing and a fitness training schedule (which we'll cover in chapters 4-7) that fits your lifestyle. Just pick what time of day works best for you to fit in your exercise, and I will help you nourish your body to maximize your results. You may want to mark this page and refer back to it after you read through the exercise portion of The PRISE Life Protocol.

TIMING CHART FOR (R)ESISTANCE AND (I)NTERVALS

Time of Day	Morning Exercise (My Top Pick)	Lunchtime Exercise	After Work Exercise	Evening Exercise (My Last Pick)
6:00 AM	WAKE-UP TIME!			
6:15 AM	Morning Muscle Maximizer (MMM)			
6:30 AM	R: 1 hour or I: 30 minutes			
9:30 AM	Morning Snack (Optional)			
NOON		R: 1 hour or I: 30 minutes		
12:30 PM	Lunch		Lunch	Lunch
1:00 PM		Lunch		
3:30 PM	Afternoon Snack (Optional)		Afternoon Snack (Optional)	Afternoon Snack (Optional)
4:00 PM		Afternoon Snack (Optional)		
5:00 PM			R: 1 hour or I: 30 minutes	
6:30 PM	Dinner		Dinner	Dinner
7:00 PM		Dinner		
9:30 PM	Bedtime Belly fat Burner (BBB)		Bedtime Belly fat Burner (BBB)	R: 1 hour or I: 30 minutes
10:00 PM		Bedtime Belly fat Burner (BBB)		Bedtime Belly fat Burner (BBB)
10:30 PM	BEDTIME. . .			

TIMING CHART FOR (S)TRETCHING AND (E)NDURANCE

Time of Day	Morning Exercise (My Top Pick)	Lunchtime Exercise	After Work Exercise	Evening Exercise (My Last Pick)
6:00 AM	WAKE-UP TIME!			
6:15 AM	S: 1 hour or E: 1-2 hours	Morning Muscle Maximizer (MMM)	Morning Muscle Maximizer (MMM)	Morning Muscle Maximizer (MMM)
8:00 AM	Morning Muscle Maximizer (MMM)			
9:30 AM		Morning Snack	Morning Snack	Morning Snack
11:00 AM	Morning Snack			
NOON		S: 1 hour or E: 1-2 hours		
12:30 PM			Lunch	Lunch
1:30 PM		Lunch		
2:00 PM	Lunch			
3:30 PM			Afternoon Snack	Afternoon Snack
5:00 PM	Afternoon Snack	Afternoon Snack	S: 1 hour or E: 1-2 hours	
6:30 PM			Dinner	Dinner
8:00 PM	Dinner	Dinner		S: 1 hour or E: 1-2 hours
9:30 PM			Bedtime Belly fat Burner (BBB)	
10:00 PM	Bedtime Belly Fat Burner (BBB)	Bedtime Belly Fat Burner (BBB)		Bedtime Belly Fat Burner (BBB)
10:30 PM	BEDTIME . . .			

THE OPTIMAL PROTEIN PACING PLAN

My original Optimal Protein Pacing plan is the basic formula followed by all the men and women in my research studies. The average American diet already consists of 50% carbs, 16% protein, and 34% fat, so we're only talking about small changes to what you eat, not a full diet overhaul. That should make this program a lot less daunting than some of the others out there. By cutting back on things like soda, candy, and simple, refined carbs and adding healthy protein from grass-fed, free-range, wild, organic animal sources (including whey protein), and organic, local, plant-based sources, as well as healthy fats to your meals, you'll get the scale to start moving in the right direction.

I want to add two other pacing strategies that you will definitely want to try to get into your daily routine as soon as possible. One is what I call the Morning Muscle Maximizer (MMM) and the other the Bedtime Belly fat Burner (BBB)! These are two more daily commitments that will assure that you get the right type of protein into your body at the right time.

Thirty years of metabolism research has taught me that starting your day with a nourishing protein-rich breakfast provides a significant health benefit, maintaining Protein Pacing meals evenly spaced throughout the day will optimize body weight control and enhance body composition, among many other health and fitness benefits, and ending your day with the right type of protein at night will keep your metabolism working even while you sleep!

Protein Pacing Meal/Snack Options (20g servings)

Key points to remember:

1) Consume at each of your four to six daily mini-meals beginning with breakfast.

2) Adjust from 20g to 40g as needed.

3) Consume immediately after exercise.

4) Consume a serving two hours prior to going to bed.

Quick Reference Guide:

Legumes (choose dry version):

Black beans, chickpeas: 8 oz. (1 cup) Kidney beans: 13.5 oz.

Lentils: 8oz (1 cup)

Nuts and seeds (unsalted, dry-roasted): Peanuts, dry roasted, unsalted: 3.5 oz. peanut butter: 5 tablespoons almonds, dry roasted, unsalted: 3.5 oz. cashews, dry roasted, unsalted: 4.5 oz. sunflower seeds: 3.5 oz.

Pumpkin seeds: 4.0 oz. flaxseed, ground: 3.5 oz. wheat germ: 2.75 oz.

Fish:

Salmon: 3.5 oz. Tilapia: 3 oz.

Haddock, halibut: 3.0 oz. cod: 3.0 oz.

Swordfish: 3.0 oz. Tuna/mackerel/ sardines in can: 3.0 oz.

Egg:

Cooked egg white: 4 eggs Hardboiled, scrambled eggs: 3 eggs Egg substitute: 7 oz.

Milk (organic):

Skim: 21 oz. (2.5 cups)

1% plain, chocolate: 20 oz. (2.5 cups)

Protein Powders and Supplements: Undenatured whey protein concentrate, isolate or hydrolysate: powders (1 scoop of 20–30 g), in meal replacement bars (range from 15–30 g per bar). Brown rice, fava, mung, legume, or pea protein (1–2 scoops of 20 g). Bone broth or collagen protein powder or liquid.

Yogurt:

Greek yogurt, plain (non-fat): 8 oz.

Greek yogurt, plain (2%): 8 oz.

Kefir, plain (low-fat): 14 oz.

Yogurt, non/low-fat, plain: 16 oz. (2 cups)

Cottage Cheese:

Non-fat cottage cheese: 5.5 oz. 1%

Low-fat cottage cheese: 6 oz.

2% Cottage cheese: 8 oz.

4% Cottage cheese: 7 oz.

Meat (choose local, free-range, grass-fed, whenever possible):

Lean beef, sirloin, buffalo: 3.5 oz. (avg. of all cuts)

Chicken breast, w/o skin: 2.5 oz.

Chicken, dark meat, w/o skin: 2.5 oz.

Sliced turkey or ham: 3.5 oz.

99% fat-free ground turkey: 3 oz.z

Turkey breast, w/o skin: 2.5 oz.

Turkey dark meat, w/o skin: 2.5 oz.

Porkchop: 3 oz.

Pork tenderloin: 3 oz.

IS BREAKFAST IMPORTANT?

There continues to be enormous media attention and controversy surrounding the topic of whether breakfast is an important meal. This topic is especially popular when parents, teachers, administrators, coaches, and children are scrambling to prepare for the start of school. Unfortunately, the truth of whether breakfast is an important start to a productive day is often missed or neglected. Despite a flurry of recent news articles suggesting that breakfast eaters are not healthier than breakfast-skippers, the science says they are. As a definition of "healthier," we mean improved body weight control and body composition management, and in some cases better brain power and mental performance.

I'm here to help you understand why there appears to be confusion over the question, "Are breakfast eaters healthier?" The answer is YES. Several recent intervention studies from our laboratory provide strong support for eating a Protein Pacing diet, especially at breakfast—to decrease total body weight and body fat (including abdominal/visceral fat), while improving heart and metabolic health.

The overwhelming conclusion of these recent studies clearly shows that a high-quality protein breakfast is indeed healthier than skipping breakfast entirely or indulging in a typical high-carbohydrate breakfast. While most of the studies have focused on weight control and body composition, a growing body of research is measuring cognitive and academic performance as well.

Therefore, the takeaway message is to start your day with a nourishing protein- and fiber-rich breakfast, fondly called the Morning Muscle Maximizer (MMM), which provides significant health and performance benefits. The strategy behind the MMM is to eat your first Protein Pacing meal within an hour of waking up. The number one reason for this is because your body is in a state of protein breakdown by the time you wake up in the morning following an overnight fast, and this is not an ideal environment to preserve and build healthy lean muscle mass. Thus, starting your day with a Protein Pacing meal to initiate protein synthesis to help maintain and start to build healthy lean muscle mass and fuel your brain is your top priority and makes the MMM one of the most important meals of the day, without question!

WHAT ABOUT EATING AT NIGHT?

Here's some great news for you! It's important to eat your last Protein Pacing meal in the evening. I encourage you to incorporate the Bedtime Belly fat Burner, which targets the most abundant site for fat storage, just beneath the surface of our skin, called subcutaneous fat.

Subcutaneous fat is found all over the body and has a tendency to accumulate in larger amounts centrally around the abdomen (belly) in men, and is referred to as android fat and given the name "apple shape." In women, subcutaneous fat deposits accumulate in greater amounts around the hips and thighs and are called gynoid fat, or "pear shape." When excess fat accumulates in the belly (android) region, some gets stored deeper and surrounds the vital organs, such as the heart, liver, kidney, and pancreas, and interferes with the normal healthy functioning of these organs. This deeper storage of fat around the vital organs is termed visceral fat and leads to significant disease risk for diabetes and heart disease, including high blood pressure, obesity-related disease, and even certain cancers.

We want to do everything in our power to get rid of this dangerous visceral "belly" fat. While men are more likely to store excess fat in the belly and, therefore, have greater visceral fat and disease risk, women of post-menopausal age are at similar risk for visceral fat accumulation and thus disease risk due to changes in hormones (lack of estrogen).

Unfortunately, given our current nutrition and food landscape around the world, more and more people are at risk of disease because of excess abdominal belly fat and visceral fat, including young boys and girls. The main reason for this disturbing public health concern is likely due to excess calorie intake, especially refined simple sugars. In fact, recent research has shown a link between higher simple sugar intake (sugar-sweetened drinks) and higher visceral fat levels in adolescents (14-18 years old).

Perhaps most alarming was the finding in those with the highest sugary-drink intake also showed the highest levels of the stress hormone cortisol upon waking in the morning. Talk about an addictive response! We are creating a toxic environment for our children by exposing them to an overabundance of sugar-sweetened drinks, which may be altering their stress hormone levels by the time they awake in the morning, all of which are associated with a significantly greater accumulation of the dangerous visceral fat. Something has to change.

The PRISE Life Protocol and especially Protein Pacing have consistently shown that the timing of when you eat protein near bedtime may have a beneficial impact on your visceral fat, and the research I've done as well as that of my colleagues over the past ten years has consistently proven that when a bedtime Protein Pacing snack is provided within two hours of going to bed, visceral fat always drops drastically. This is exactly why I want you to start to incorporate this tonight. Don't delay!

I hope you now agree that the science of eating breakfast with protein and a protein snack at bedtime are truly Protein Pacing maximizers to your overall PRISE Life Protocol. You really can start to get rid of the dangerous visceral fat and start to feel better. You may even wake up feeling more refreshed than you have in years. You will feel great and be on top of your game!

SAMPLE PROTEIN PACING MEAL PLAN

MEAL	FOODS
Morning Muscle Maximizer (Breakfast) 20–40g of Protein	Choice of: Shakes, Smoothies, Pancakes, Waffles, Muffins, or Bowls with fresh fruits and veggies: Multivitamin with adaptogens and antioxidants
Mid-morning Snack (Optional) 20–40g of Protein	Choice of: Bowls with grains, nuts, seeds, fruit, veggies, dark chocolate; Bars, Shakes, or Smoothies: Optional; Natural-sourced caffeine beverage with antioxidants and adaptogens
Lunch 20–40g of Protein	Choice of: Shakes or Smoothies; Fish, Poultry, Beef, or Pork (grass-fed, wild, free-range); Legumes and Grains (quinoa, millet, amaranth, brown/wild rice, etc.). All with fresh veggies and fruits
Mid-afternoon Snack (Optional) 20–40g of Protein	Choice of: Bowls with grains, nuts, seeds, fruit, veggies, dark chocolate; Bars, Shakes, or Smoothies: Optional; Natural-sourced caffeine beverage with antioxidants and adaptogens
Dinner 20–40g of Protein Bedtime Belly Fat Burner (Evening Snack) 20–40g of Protein	Choice of: Fish, Poultry, Beef, Pork (grass-fed, wild, free-range); Legumes and Grains (quinoa, millet, amaranth, brown/wild rice). All with fresh veggies and fruits
	Choice of: Shakes, Bars, Smoothies or Puddings with fresh or powdered veggies, fruits, and nuts/seeds. Add Dr. Paul's Sleeping Aids of magnesium, calcium, vitamin D, tart cherry juice, pumpkin seeds, melatonin, valerian root, and air-mist of lavender oil

*Drink plain water and with electrolytes throughout the day. Shakes/Bars/Smoothies/Pancakes/Waffles include either animal and/or plant-based protein sources (whole foods and powders) such as; undenatured whey, egg, pea, fava, mung, brown rice, pumpkin, collagen, etc. Bowls include probiotics and may be either animal and/or plant-based sources from dairy, almonds, cashews, flax, pea, quinoa, oats, cassava root, tapioca, chia, locust bean, hemp, coconut.

For some people, combining my Protein Pacing with any of the diet plans I list above may result in even more dramatic improvement in body composition. It can be adapted to any healthy diet plan and boost your results to the next level. By incorporating the Protein Pacing plan with your nutrition/diet plan of choice (such as a plant-based, Mediterranean, Paleo, fat-adapted/ketogenic diet), you may find that you have greater energy, a decreased desire for unhealthy food, improved mood, and greatly improved body composition. Combined with the metabolic increase, greater satiety, and improved protein synthesis you will gain from the Protein Pacing plan, you can take your lifestyle to the next level of performance.

PROTEIN PACING WITH A KETOGENIC DIET

After I created the original plan, I became interested in the recent trends in fat-adapted or ketogenic-eating strategies. So, what does it mean to be "fat adapted?" As it turns out, humans have been around for quite a long time, much longer than cookies, cake, bread, soda, and all of the other high-carbohydrate, refined, and starchy foods that many of us love so much. How did humans survive for thousands of years without pasta and all of its starchy compadres? It's coming to light that a large majority of the human diet was historically made up of plant and animal protein and fats, along with whatever vegetables, nuts, seeds, and berries were in season and naturally occurring.

How diets have evolved from when humans were first hunter-gatherers is what has given the Paleo diet traction today. A ketogenic or fat-adapted diet may seem extreme, and indeed it is night and day in comparison to the foods that many of us choose to eat on a daily basis, but a diet with the right types and amounts of fats can help you to unlock the full energy potential of all of your stored fat! Imagine: You have the potential to feel consistently satiated while also getting rid of all of your unnecessary body fat at the same time!

With a fat-adapted diet, you can train your metabolism to use fat as the primary energy source. This means that even while at rest and exercising at moderate intensity, you will be primarily burning fat as fuel. Recent scientific research on "thinking evolutionary" when it comes to dieting has even demonstrated that higher-fat diets have the potential to turn on aspects of the human genome, stored within us, that help us to burn and utilize greater proportions of fat on our body and in our diets, the way our ancestors did.

A fat-adapted diet is generally comprised of 60%–70% fat, sourced from healthy saturated and monounsaturated fats. The rest of your dietary needs are satisfied by healthy proteins (from plants as well as healthy and well-cared-for animals that have the benefit of containing delicious and healthy fats as well) using my Protein Pacing plan (~20%) and minimal carbs. The carbs that you do eat will comprise 10%–15% of your dietary intake and will be largely resistant starch and nutrient-dense vegetables and greens. The difference and speed at which body fat is released may be truly exceptional.

While it is exciting to see the extra effect the fat-adapted ketogenic diet offers, it remains controversial for many experts, so proceed with caution. Regardless, you have to follow those basics about the use of my Protein Pacing plan whether you choose the fat-adapted, plant-based, Mediterranean, MIND, WW (formerly Weight Watchers), Atkins, Paleolithic, or any other diet.

PROTEIN PACING IS NOT A HIGH-PROTEIN DIET

To be clear, Protein Pacing is NOT a high-protein diet. As I stated earlier, it's the right type and amount of protein at the right time. And don't be fooled by all those posers who claim we are eating too much protein; in fact, just the opposite is true. Remember that well-respected and validated scientific data I shared? As the worldwide obesity epidemic has ballooned since the 1980s, data shows we are eating too many carbohydrates, especially simple sugars, during this same time period, and protein intake has decreased!

Thus, Protein Pacing holds the key to healthy weight loss and optimal performance. Of course, it would be amazing to eat healthy and tasty protein foods throughout the day. But the reality is, many of us do not have the time, energy, or money to prepare and purchase these foods for every meal we eat; that would be a full-time job!

Instead, I recommend combining high-quality whole foods with nutrient-dense protein powders and bars to maximize the Protein Pacing plan effects, and, you guessed it, I have the science to back it up.

For example, sound science has proven that four to six meals per day containing 20–40g of protein per meal from protein-rich plant and animal foods and powders and bars (such as naturally sourced undenatured whey and plant-based protein shakes and bars) stimulates metabolism up to eight times more than fat and two-and-a-half times more than carbs; optimizes protein synthesis needed for enhanced repair and building of lean muscle mass, and quenches hunger better than any other nutrient. All of this helps maintain an ideal body composition, leading to optimal health and peak performance. Here is a chart that shares some ideas of what protein to use.

An easy way to keep track of your Protein Pacing plan each time you eat a meal or snack is to use the palm of your hand as the serving size for any animal-based products such as beef, chicken, turkey, fish, eggs; the size of your fist for a plant-based protein serving such as quinoa, chickpeas, tofu, legumes, and lentils; and one to two scoops of undenatured whey or plant-based powders in the form of brown rice, bean (fava, mung, etc) and pea protein.

TRAVEL AND PROTEIN PACING

My first introduction to what I now call a Road Warrior (RW) occurred during my childhood while watching my dad, a traveling clothes salesman, prepare for the workweek every Sunday. His routine involved organizing and packing huge bags of clothing samples he would carry up from the basement, one by one, and loading them into the trunk of his car.

It was an exhausting way to start the workweek, and it didn't stop there. Every day during the week he would go through the same routine along his route, unloading and loading each sample clothing bag at each of the department stores and private retail shops he visited. At the time, I didn't pay much attention to the physical demands of his job as a traveling salesman. But now, I fully appreciate what he accomplished each week for more than 33 years!

Without question, it was his Protein Pacing diet (OK, and bag lifting) that kept him healthy, strong, and mentally prepared throughout his career as a true RW. Similarly, many hardworking men and women continue to hit the pavement, train tracks, or airways as RWs, and a healthy, nourishing diet is crucial to keeping them on their A-game when they reach their destination.

I hate to say it, but one of the largest barriers to being successful in a lifestyle routine is consistency, even while we are on the run or living our hectic lives. It's important to think and plan ahead and figure out ways to always have nourishment at our fingertips when we are running errands, working at the office, or in places that are not conducive to healthy eating. Once we get into the habit, it will become second nature to be prepared.

I hope this little story helps you relate and want to be with the best of the RWs—prepared and ready to take on a healthy life!

To help you, here are some strategies I put together to provide the necessary foundation:

4 PROTEIN PACING RULES FOR ROAD WARRIORS

1 Eat a protein- and fiber-rich breakfast. Starting the day with a 20–40g serving of protein and 8–10g of fiber revs your metabolism, quenches hunger, and promotes healthy lean body mass (muscles). Other added benefits are increased mental focus and staying regular.

2 Eat 20–40g of protein at each of your meals, especially important during your "power lunches" to keep you mentally sharp and energized. Too often, poor food choices at lunch turn "power lunches" into "weakness lunches," and we feel sluggish and energy depleted.

This protein stabilizes blood sugar, replenishes energy stores, nourishes muscles and the brain, and revs metabolism. Plan to eat 0.7–0.85g of protein per pound of body weight per day. Most packaging on food contains this information.

For example:

A 150-pound person should eat 105–128g of protein per day (150 x 0.7 = 105g; 150 x 0.85 = 128g).

*If you add exercise to your daily routine, add an additional 20–25g immediately following your exercise session. Individuals over sixty years of age should aim for a higher level of protein intake (0.85g per pound of body weight).

3 Pack a cooler. Stuff the cooler with water, cut veggies, fresh fruit, Greek yogurt, cottage cheese, homemade protein smoothies, natural peanut butter with rice cakes, homemade hummus, trail mix, hard-boiled eggs, protein bars, and your favorite stuffed pita or sandwich wraps. If nothing else, it keeps hunger pangs in check and drastically reduces the likelihood of your binging on fast food.

If you plan to be driving all day, restock the cooler at a grocery store along the way. This also provides an opportunity to get out of the car, stretch, walk around, and pick the food you want, instead of sitting at a restaurant or, worse yet, a fast-food drive-up window and ordering only what is available on the menu. I highly recommend grocery store pit stops en route to your destination.

It's more difficult to restock at a grocery store when traveling by train, so plan ahead and pack some extra protein bars. Your goal is to feel nourished and energized, and thinking clearly when you arrive at your destination.

4 Eat Protein Pacing every three to four hours with the last serving within two hours of going to bed at night. I recommend traveling with a protein bar (providing ~20–30g of protein) or protein powder (24–36g) to mix with water whenever hunger strikes.

Flying is often the most time-efficient travel method and allows us to arrive at our destination the quickest, but it's also the trickiest environment to maintain a healthy eating plan. Restrictions on the size of carry-ons make bringing food a challenge. This is unfortunate because air travel food (airports and planes) often suffers in taste and quality.

Regardless, packing food for air travel is the same—think higher protein, nutrient-dense, and convenience. Excellent choices are protein bars, powders, and homemade trail mix. During the flight, choose fresh veggies and hummus, and fruit with nuts, yogurt, and trail mix, and always opt for water or tea to drink.

FOR THE LOVE OF FATS

Now that we've thoroughly covered Protein Pacing, let's talk about fats. Remember how I mentioned fat-adapted Protein Pacing may allow even more chances to lose weight and grow lean muscle? Well, I am referring to specific and healthy types of fats.

Here is a general breakdown of the fats to love, and where to find them:

Specific saturated fats: Highly stable, largely nonreactive molecules with a good shelf life. These are generally solid at room temperature.

- Butter from grass-fed cows: An excellent source of fat-soluble vitamins A, D, and K, butter from certified 100% grass-fed cows is not always available year-round but can be recognized by the distinctive golden yellow color obtained through the presence of naturally occurring beta-carotene, a powerful antioxidant. Butter from grass-fed cows also contains conjugated-linoleic acid (CLA), which may have anti-cancer properties. Short-chain fatty acids are easily and quickly absorbed through the gastrointestinal tract, where they are immediately metabolized for energy in healthy active people.
- Coconut oil: Largely made up of short- and medium-chain fatty acids. It can be kept at room temperature for a long time without rancidity.
- Lauric acid: Found in cow and goat milk, palm kernel oil. Limit to 10-20g per day.

Monounsaturated fats: These fats are found in foods like almonds, olive oil, and avocados. They are slightly less stable than saturated fats, and so are often liquid at room temperature.

Polyunsaturated fats: These fats are generally considered the most unstable. They are made up of long carbon chains that do not stack together well. This means they are often liquid even below room temperature. These oils are susceptible to spoilage (rancidity) and can easily burn or oxidize when used as a cooking agent. For this reason, it's usually not a good idea to use polyunsaturated fats while cooking.

THE MAGIC OF COOKING AT HOME

Finally, never forget grandma's cooking. Remember how nice it was to sit around the family table and enjoy food that was cooked with love and have conversations with those you cared about? Food is nourishment for the body and the soul.

That is why I encourage you to eat home-cooked food that is organic and grown locally whenever possible. Shopping for, preparing, and cooking your own food is one easy way to cut calories. Even at restaurants, a lot of the foods you eat are prepackaged and just heated up. True cooking is hard to come by outside of your kitchen, but it's important if you want to know what's actually going into your body.

What's wrong with packaged foods? A lot! Did you know that packaged foods are actually manufactured to make you feel hungrier after eating them? Most processed foods contain the "big three": lots of fat, sugar, and salt, all of which trigger your hunger at warp speed. Processed foods are designed in big laboratories with the intention of making it so that the more you eat, the more you want to eat. This happens because the foods are missing vital nutrients your body needs. By swapping out a bag of chips for a snack of an apple with nut or seed butter, you'll feel full for much longer without taking in any extra calories.

How do you do it when you're pressed for time? It's all about planning. My wife and I raised our three boys on home-cooked meals by making up a new menu each week and doing shopping and prep on the weekend, before homework and sports practices kicked into high gear. If chili was on the menu, I'd pre-chop all of my veggies as soon as I got home from the store. If it was taco night, my wife would cook up extra ground turkey to be used in the next night's marinara sauce. Look for ways to get ahead, and cooking will feel a lot more manageable.

Also, don't be afraid of using healthy packaged foods like canned tomatoes or beans or frozen spinach and even protein powders (undenatured whey and plant-based) to add to baked goods, casseroles, soups or as on-the-go meals. Take advantage of nutrient-dense engineered foods that come in the form of protein powders, bars, and snacks. I've used these extensively in my research, showing phenomenal benefit. If you can swap in a few pre-cut, or pre-cooked ingredients into an otherwise fresh meal, I'm all for it!

EATING PLUS EXERCISE

Study after study shows that eating the right foods at the right time can actually make you less hungry and that people who work out the right way tend to eat less afterward than those who stay on the couch or who exercise the wrong way. But if you find the opposite to be true—that you want to scarf down pretty much anything in sight after exercise—you're not alone. Many people who begin to exercise also increase food intake. This can sabotage your best diet and healthy eating efforts. If you find yourself wanting to do this, ask yourself why.

Did you eat a mini protein-packed meal before exercise? If not, chances are you will feel famished when you're done. Did you participate in an intense cycling class? If so, you may be telling yourself that you "deserve" to take in a few hundred extra calories after all the ones you just burned off. Or if all you do is endurance/aerobic exercise every day hour after hour, your hunger cues will scream for food, and lots of it, all the time! Exercise is not a free pass to eat freely and without consequence. If you find this starting to happen, ease off on your exercise for a week until you really get the eating routine down. Once your body and brain know you're taking in more than enough food to fuel your day, add exercise back in. But make sure it's the right exercise, in this case, The PRISE Life fitness routine!

Each time you exercise is an opportunity to build a little more muscle (or a lot if you're Protein Pacing and doing the RISE fitness!). Adding more muscle to your frame is one easy way to burn more calories all day. Studies have shown that adding more muscle can help your body burn hundreds of extra calories a day, especially fat calories. That means you'll be burning more calories every day—even the days you take off from exercise. Best of all, the more fit you are, the more your lean muscle prefers to get energy from your body fat over any other fuel source.

There's more. Exercise is a proven antidote for stress and anxiety. If you're feeling stressed about work or your home life, you may find you want to sneak in more cookies and chips. (Emotional eating is rarely about overindulging because you're just so happy!) By managing these feelings in healthier ways— through my Stretching and Endurance exercise— you'll save yourself all those unwanted calories while tapping into your fat stores for fuel. It's a win-win situation. Finally, committing to an exercise routine makes it easier to stick to an eating plan. There's a lot of science to back this up, but you may have noticed it on your own.

When you're able to accomplish one goal, it makes the other ones seem even more within reach. If you start your day with a brisk walk around the neighborhood, you may be less likely to reach for a pastry for breakfast. If you sign up for a fitness class after work, you may be more mindful throughout the day about putting food in your belly that will fuel you instead of exhaust you. If you do decide to splurge on the occasional ice cream cone or a candy bar, you'll know exactly how to zap it away—with exercise. This is the synchronicity of using true nourishment with proper amounts of smart exercise to attain optimal health!

Please take it from me; I've developed my PRISE Life Protocol to help you take the road less traveled to optimal health and peak performance because I've done the research for you!

One additional point I want to leave you with: I have some exciting new research I will be sharing with all of you very soon regarding the effects of my Protein Pacing and PRISE Life Protocol on enhancing your mood—so stay tuned!

FINAL TIPS FROM DR. PAUL

1 **Pay attention to what your body is telling you (listen to body cues).**

As I've highlighted numerous times in the book, counting and measuring your calories is not nearly as healthy and beneficial for your overall health as the quality and timing of your calories. In other words, the quality of your calories always reigns supreme over the number of calories for optimal health and peak performance. With this in mind, the number one question I'm bombarded with on a daily basis from my followers and others is, "Which specific nutrition plan (diet) should I be following for the best results?" My answer is always the same: The best nutrition plan is the one your body tells you to eat!

Our bodies are programmed for homeostasis, which means a state of equilibrium among cellular and overall physiological processes that maintain a balanced resting state. When things are "off" in our bodies, signals are sent from our cells, tissues, organs, etc., to our brain in an attempt to correct the problem. Many call this "self-regulation," and the top performers in the world do this better than everyone else. They are masters of self-regulating and getting things back in order as quickly as possible. Within the context of optimal nourishment for health and performance, the same thing happens. If we are depleted of essential nutrients, our bodies will send warning signals to the brain to increase our intake of those nutrients. One nutrient that is a top priority every day is our protein stores, because proteins are involved in every cellular process of the body and can never be compromised. This is why Protein Pacing is a necessity and foundation for EVERY type of diet and nutrition plan. But when it comes to fats and carbs, they can wax and wane on a daily basis, depending on the needs of the body (cells).

❷ Understand your cravings

If you crave carb-loaded foods, this means you may be lacking in vitamins, minerals, and fiber, and therefore should increase your intake of fresh vegetables, fruits, legumes (beans), and whole grains.

If you are craving fatty foods, you're probably exhausted (physically and emotionally), you may be more prone to sickness, and need the additional calories from foods like avocados, nuts, seeds, and oils (coconut, olive, etc.) to help replenish your energy stores and fuel your nervous and immune systems, which depends on a healthy dose of essential fats/lipids (fatty acids) for optimal function.

❸ Eat more often with Protein Pacing

I'll repeat it one last time: Eating at timed intervals throughout the day burns more calories than aiming for three square meals. Keep your metabolism revved continuously with Protein Pacing meals. You can do this by paying attention to the amount and type of protein foods you're eating and how you're spacing your meals throughout the day. The goal from this style of eating is to provide the body with the ideal amount and type of high-quality protein to fuel the cells of the body so they can maximize the pathway of protein synthesis every four hours instead of overloading your system with too large a load of protein with just a few meals a day.

If weight loss is your goal, you may find it's easiest to simply cut your current meals in half— literally—eating one half in one sitting and the other half a few hours later but making sure your protein intake is at the critical amount of 20–40g. I usually advise people to eat four to six times a day.

If you've been worried that eating more often might spell trouble for your diet, think again. One of my favorite things about this pacing approach is that you're less likely to give in to cravings. Research shows you feel fuller on small, frequent protein-balanced meals than after eating a few big meals. When you actually plan in these small and frequent protein-pacing food breaks, you're much less likely to eat off-script and eat unhealthy things. And there's one more benefit to smaller portions spaced out throughout the day: no more bloat or feeling of being stuffed!

❹ Incorporate the Bedtime Bellyfat Burner

My mother used to say that no good things ever happen after midnight. With eating, I'd venture it's more like 8:00 p.m. Setting this cutoff for yourself will eliminate the calories that come from late-night crunching and munching, and it'll give your metabolism a chance to really rest before the next day. Plus, the calories you eat at night are more likely to be stored as fat rather than burned off, so limit your intake after dinner to my Bedtime Bellyfat Burner (BBB) plan, which is the last snack of the day. This is one of the most important snacks of the day because it provides a high-quality protein feeding during the overnight time period, which feeds your muscles so you can burn fat and support your lean muscle mass throughout the night. How does this sound? You can have an occasional glass of wine or beer with your evening meal if you like, but switch to water or herbal tea after that. But no matter what, make the last calories you eat a Protein Pacing snack of 20–30g of high-quality protein. The BBB is also essential for athletes and fitness-enthusiasts to replenish energy stores for training and competition the next day.

⑤ Dish out more Low-Energy, Nutrient-Dense (LEND) foods

Protein isn't the only thing I want you to eat more of. High fiber should also be on the list. These are foods that are filling without being heavy. They can help you get the nutrients you need to stay healthy and strong, but they won't make you pack on pounds. In fact, they'll do just the opposite. You can eat a plateful of these low-energy, nutrient-dense (LEND) foods and lose weight because they're not full of calories. The LEND foods will supply vitamins, minerals, fiber, and special nutrients called phytochemicals (plant chemicals), which fight disease and increase energy levels but don't carry a high caloric cost.

LEND foods tend to be high in fiber, which keeps you regular, lowers cholesterol, maintains blood sugar levels, and can make you feel full. Just like protein, these LEND foods require more energy to digest and metabolize than a lot of other foods. That means you can eat more without worrying about those bites sticking to your belly, hips, and thighs.

If you've been worried that the Protein Pacing plan will tell you to eat plain chicken breasts all day long, my LEND list will put those fears to rest. All plant-based foods such as green and rainbow-colored fresh vegetables and fruits are LEND foods, and so are legumes, such as lentils, split peas, chickpeas, black beans, and kidney beans. You can also go nuts over nuts and seeds like chia, pumpkin (pepitas), and flaxseed and whole grains such as quinoa, oats, barley, and rice. I've already talked about protein-rich animal and plant foods, and they're on the LEND list too.

Having shared all of the above, I want to make sure I tell you that there is some truth to those additional calories, and here is my tip that gets me as close to a dieting plan as I feel comfortable with:

❻ Shave off surplus calories

So, just how much of these foods do you get to eat? If your goal is weight loss and you're into calorie counting, I'd aim for about 1,200–1,400 calories a day for women and 1,500–1,800 calories a day for men. Right now, you may eat only a few hundred calories more than this, consuming more like 1,800–2,000 calories a day. Stopping at 1,200–1,800 calories will be easy if you follow my five other tips.

Keep in mind, I don't want you to ever feel hungry or deprived. You may eat the same volume of food—or an even greater amount—but the foods you eat will have more metabolically active nutrients (protein), fiber and fewer calories in them. You may go from eating a few slices of pizza to eating a salad with chicken and a side of hummus and pita. Your belly will be happy, but you won't be storing all those excess calories as fat. If you have pounds to lose, it's an indication that you may have been eating the wrong amount and type of food at the wrong time for your body to burn calories and instead stored those extra calories in your trouble zones— usually the hips, thighs, and belly.

Once you've mastered this style of eating, you might want to try cutting out more surplus calories. In some of my recent studies, when women and men followed this same eating plan just at 1,200 and 1,500 calories a day, respectively, weight loss results skyrocketed to an average of twenty-five pounds in eleven weeks. Of course, if you're in a hurry to meet your weight-loss goals, you can jump right in and start here.

You already have the tools—the LEND list, the Protein Pacing, the reduction of processed foods and carbohydrates—so follow the diet at the calorie count that best serves you and be sure to download The PRISE Life app today and use it as your guide to successfully pacing your meals throughout the day.

In general, eating slightly more calories of healthier food from a better source is always better than feeling deprived and seeking refuge in processed food. Give yourself some slack during your dietary transition if times get tough and you start to feel hungry. Fat- and protein-dense snacks such as avocado with some wild fish or slices of free-range chicken or a protein shake/smoothie or bar can help to signal satiety and decrease any sugar cravings you may be having—a worthy goal, even if it means you eat more calories than usual for that day.

Thomas Edison could not have been more accurate when he stated, "The doctor of the future will no longer treat the human frame with drugs, but rather will cure and prevent disease with nutrition and food." It's time for us to step into and embrace this future.

CHAPTER 4
(R) IS FOR RESISTANCE

Dr. Paul says: "Resistance helps you
burn more fat and gain more muscle!"

PROTEIN PACING | **RESISTANCE** | INTERVAL | STRETCHING | ENDURANCE

It's time to RISE up and get moving. The next four chapters will guide you through the RISE portion of The PRISE Life. They all are crucial components to an overall healthy life, and don't worry, it'll be easy and fun. Remember when I told you how busy my wife and I were with our three young sons and hectic professional lives? This exercise routine was developed to work perfectly for busy people like you. I have road-tested it in the lab with human subjects, on my own body, and with hundreds of thousands of people just like you, and I can assure you that with just a small commitment of time—three to four hours weekly—you can see dramatic results when you pair the RISE fitness strategy with the Protein Pacing eating plan we outlined in Chapter 3. Ready? Let's go!

It is finally time to tackle the topic that scares most people…: Exercise. This is why I will use the word fitness instead because it has a much more positive connotation. The great news is that fitness no longer needs to be a burden. First, because you see how the protein-pacing lifestyle program is effective even without fitness. Second, because throughout this RISE journey you have control and you get to choose what you like to do; therefore, it can actually be fun!

BUSTING COMMON EXERCISE MYTHS

In the studies I performed, you may have noticed that I did not make fitness a requirement. That was intentional. I wanted to be sure we could gather true statistics. But in real life, fitness is necessary. The good news is, you don't have to do as much as you have been led to believe or work as strenuously as you may have been told. Everything I teach will help you build lean muscle and get rid of harmful belly fat, especially that dangerous visceral fat.

I know that anyone starting a new fitness program wants all the hard work and sweat to pay off in some way. Some of the more common payoffs include weight and fat loss, toned muscles, increased energy, improved mood, and better athletic performance. However, the statistics tell us that most people who begin a fitness program don't receive these payoffs.

❶ Working out hard every day is good for you

The truth is, we should be physically active every day, but we should NOT "work out" every day. Recently, I came across a statistic showing that more than 60% of Americans make New Year's resolutions, mostly to get healthier (>85%), but only 8% are successful in achieving their resolutions. Why is this? How can so many well-intentioned and determined people fail at such a noble, worthwhile, and healthy cause? We have an abundance of easily accessible information on how to get fit, eat well, and manage our stress, so it's not a result of not knowing what or how to do it.

Many current fitness programs are to blame for this high failure rate because they are too intense and time-consuming and hold us hostage by expecting us to work out like a fitness-aholic nearly every day of the week! None of us, including top athletes, should be pushing ourselves to the brink of physical exhaustion every day thinking that it is the only way to achieve fitness, health, and wellness. While you may experience a few positive results in the short term, it does little, if anything, to keep you motivated in the long term. In fact, it does the opposite. It creates the perfect situation for injury and burnout. By following The PRISE Life, you add four days of fun fitness to your weekly routine, and on the other days you stay physically active by walking, gardening, shopping, cleaning the house, etc. It's the perfect balance of fitness and activity so you feel energized all the time.

❷ Everyone should know what to do already

In my experience, working with tens of thousands of people on a regular basis of all ages, fitness levels, and health statuses, the most common complaint I hear on their quest to become healthier is, "I don't know what to do or how to do it!" In other words, despite the massive amount of fitness information we have at our fingertips, most of us struggle to make sense of it or have a clear understanding of what steps to take. It has become a case of "(mis)-information overload" that has created confusion, frustration, and an epidemic of inaction, and has had the opposite effect of what it was designed to prevent—poor eating habits, physical inactivity, stress, and disease.

THE ACRONYM PRISE

As you can see, PRISE is an acronym, the "P" for Protein Pacing and the "RISE" exercise portion, which I will define below. The entire PRISE Protocol is synergistic and works perfectly when you implement the four exercise components together. It trains your muscles, lungs, heart, and mind, turning your body into an even more efficient fuel-burning machine. The workouts are all under an hour, except Endurance (one-plus hours), and you only have to fit in each workout once a week. That means that four hours of exercise a week can help you double—or triple— your weight-loss results!

To accelerate your results and firm as you burn, you'll combine Protein Pacing with my signature exercise series, RISE, which helped dieters in my studies lose more weight more quickly. It preserved their lean muscle mass as well as enhanced performance outcomes among already super-fit women and men. The best part of PRISE is that it's individually tailored to your own personal health and fitness goals to ensure you achieve maximal results in the quickest time possible. Because it's so easily customized to each person, it's not uncommon for an eighty-seven-year-old woman to perform a PRISE exercise routine alongside a twenty-four-year-old world-class athlete! That is an exercise program with longevity!

PRISE is revolutionizing how the scientific and medical community prescribes and recommends exercise to the entire population, and is the change agent we've all been looking for to finally make an impact on the epidemic of obesity and lifestyle-related diseases, but also to create the next wave of world-class athletes.

RISE STANDS FOR:

(R)esistance exercise —Resistance training includes traditional strength training, of course, but also more functional resistance exercises that use only your bodyweight or the addition of rubber bands, tubes, physioballs, medicine balls, and other mobile strength-training devices. It involves contracting your muscles against a force and is the best method to increase muscular function, strength, power, and endurance.

(I)nterval exercise Interval training includes specific types of short bouts of quick and intense movement of your larger muscles, with recovery periods in between. It is the best form of fitness training to develop a lean, sculpted body and to increase lean muscle mass and decrease fat mass (total and abdominal), as well as improve heart and metabolic health and fitness.

(S)tretching   Stretching training involves all types of stretches and poses (yoga, tai chi, pilates, qigong, etc.) that enhance blood flow and is the most effective fitness training to increase your muscle/tendon flexibility, joint mobility, and create a deeper mind-body connection.

(E)ndurance   Endurance training includes all the different exercises that keep your heart and muscles pumping for long periods of time in a full-body rhythmical manner to produce the greatest cardiovascular health benefits and feelings of euphoria, happiness, and mental function (executive function, decision-making, etc.).

I will show you how to perform each of these different but highly beneficial fitness training routines to give you the greatest opportunity to achieve optimal health and peak performance in the most time-efficient manner possible. There is no arguing the scientific proof I've established supporting The PRISE Life Protocol to produce amazing results in people of all ages, health, and states of fitness.

SAMPLE PRISE LIFE PROTOCOL FOR A WEEK:

Sunday	Monday	Tuesday	Wednesday	Thursday	Friday	Saturday or Sunday
Protein Pacing Every Day						
-	**R**ESISTANCE	-	**I**NTERVAL	-	**S**TRETCHING	**E**NDURANCE

Another schedule I've recommended that also includes intermittent fasting looks something like this:

Follow the Protein Pacing eating schedule Monday through Saturday and include the RISE exercise routines as prescribed below. Sunday is a day of rest both for your body and your digestion.

Monday = Resistance

Tuesday = Recovery

Wednesday = Intervals

Thursday = Stretching

Friday = Recovery

Saturday = Endurance

Sunday = Recovery (intermittent fasting)

5 STEPS BEFORE YOU BEGIN YOUR PRISE PROGRAM

It would be great if I could personally assess your level of fitness and give you the perfect plan for your body, but my PRISE Life App is the closest thing to this, so please download it now. Also, I will be hosting PRISE Life Retreats throughout the year for you to attend, so keep your eyes open for these. However, there are certain steps you can take to be sure you get the most satisfactory results from your PRISE Life fitness plan, and I recommend you do five of them before you start.

1 Obtain clearance from your health-care professional to begin participating in a fitness program. Nearly all of them will be thrilled to support you on this mission!

2 Choose an appropriate exercise intensity to avoid injury.

If you're going to take the time to exercise, you want to get the biggest payoff possible. That means finding the intensity level that is best for you, whether it's finding the right amount of weight to lift or the perfect speed to walk or run. If you don't push yourself enough, you won't make the gains you want. You will build muscle and zap calories, but not as quickly as you otherwise could.

If you go too hard, you risk injuring yourself and having to quit your fitness plan for a few workouts or even several weeks. For this reason, I have developed Dr. Paul's PRISE Intensity Scale for Fitness to help you perform the fitness routines at a level that is safe and effective for improving health and performance.

3 Choose appropriate dynamic warmup and cool-down exercises.

Many doing exercise ignore the warm-up and cool-down portion of a workout. But both are essential. A proper warm-up heats your body so it's ready to move the way you want it to. A proper cool-down stretches out some of the muscles you just challenged, making you ready for your next session. A warm-up should be active, including walking and movements such as leg and arm swings and circles. A cool-down can be active and static, including a cool-down walk and stretches such as toe touches and quad stretches. Aim to add five to ten minutes of warming and cooling activity at the front and back end of all of your workouts.

I always recommend that before starting each RISE exercise routine, you perform a walk/jog warm-up for five minutes at a moderate pace (Intensity Level 4–5). I have included a complete listing of Dynamic Warm-up exercises on The PRISE Life app and I have developed recommended exercises with explanations that are easy to follow. By following these routines, it will be easier for you to create a core program that becomes second nature versus reinventing the wheel. See step 4.

4 Download the free PRISE Life companion app to be your guide.

Now that you have clearance from your health-care professional and you understand the intensity scale and the importance of a proper warm-up and cool-down, I want to be your guide. I understand that working out alone can be challenging, so I developed The PRISE Life app. This is as close as I can get to coaching you every day. I have created video tutorials to follow and you will have a customized Protein Pacing plan loaded in that is created just for you!

5 Remember fitness is a habit and it can be fun!

Now that you're ready to go, I want to share some additional suggestions for lasting success if you have not made fitness a habit and are trying to get back into it. There are some basic guidelines that will help you decide to become fit, especially if you are on the fence or find you just need one little excuse ("Oh, gee I forgot my lucky workout shirt in the dryer!") to bow out. We've all experienced that! These steps may seem simple, but you would be surprised how using them will get you in the mood to succeed!

DR. PAUL'S PRISE INTENSITY SCALE FOR FITNESS

Dr. Paul's PRISE Intensity Scale for Fitness is an effective solution to help you choose the proper exercise intensity to reduce your risk for injury, and enjoy the results of your RISE fitness program! This scale will serve as a helpful guide when performing the RISE fitness routines. I encourage you to use the scale on your own for the next month but aim for a level of 4–6. Then, as you progress, you can slowly work to increase the intensity level at a safe pace.

INTENSITY LEVEL	DESCRIPTION	EXAMPLE
1	No Physical Movement	Seated or standing in a relaxed position.
2	Very Easy Physical Activity	Stroll pace or window shopping. Talking is easy and you are not out of breath.
3	Easy Physical Activity	A comfortable walk to a destination and able to carry a conversation. You are relaxed and not physically stressed.

4	Low Physical Activity	A brisk walk at a pace you can carry on a conversation but need to pause occasionally to catch your breath. Your heart is beating quicker and you're breathing a little deeper.
5	Low-Moderate Physical Activity	Any activity that increases your heart rate, breathing, and body temperature. You can talk but need to focus on breathing more often with effort. You could maintain this pace for hours, such as during an easy hike.
6	Moderate Physical Activity	Moderate-paced activity that starts you sweating, breathing deeper, and increasing your heart rate. You can talk but it takes effort. You could maintain this pace for hours, such as a moderate hike.
7	Moderate-Vigorous Physical Activity	A moderate-vigorous activity that gets you sweating and breathing hard and your heart rate is beating faster. You can only talk during your exhalation. You could maintain this pace up to 2–4 hours, maximum.
8	Vigorous Physical Activity	Faster-paced activity that gets you sweating, breathing hard, and your heart rate is fast. Talking is difficult. You could only maintain for 30–60 minutes, if you really push.
9	Very Vigorous Physical Activity	A near maximum activity effort. You are not able to talk and can only maintain this up to several minutes with your best effort.
10	All-out Burst of Physical Activity	A maximal physical effort, you're breathing as fast as you can, and your heart rate is at its max. You can only maintain this pace up to a minute with full effort. Only grunting and gasping at this level.

DR. PAUL'S FITNESS TIPS

Before you start PRISE, please download The PRISE Life app so you can take it with you anywhere, anytime to guarantee success! I know I said this before, but it's free and it's so important to be sure you're following the program for maximum results. Just search the app store for "PRISE Life" and look for the logo that is on the front cover of this book. And here are a few additional tips to help you get started and avoid excuses, which will likely creep in to try to sabotage your new healthy PRISE lifestyle.

Prepare ahead to avoid any excuse. Some people keep spare clothes in the car or put them by the front door, so they don't have to search for a swimsuit or exercise shoes or a towel or yoga mat. Keep your RISE commitment right where you can see it! It will not only to remind you to exercise, but will help you lose the excuses as to why you can't exercise today.

Schedule your workouts.   To get the benefits of fitness, you actually have to do it. If you're like most people I know, fitness is the first thing to fall off when your schedule gets full. But if you block it out in your calendar, this is less likely to happen. You can also recruit a workout buddy, and use your PRISE Life app, to keep you on track. When your alarm rings at 6:00 a.m., you may want to hit snooze. But if you know your friend is waiting for you at the park or gym, you'll be a lot more likely to get up and go.

Fuel and hydrate right.   What you eat and drink throughout the day will either sabotage or boost your response to fitness. *Remember . . . what you eat always exceeds any amount of fitness you do.* The goal is to have your food and drink intake and your RISE fitness plan working synergistically, not against one another. Within one hour of starting your fitness routine, plan to drink 8–16 oz. of water. (This will help you stay hydrated, even if you sweat a lot.) Also, be sure you eat something within two or three hours of starting. A small meal (think 200–300 cal.) of fresh vegetables or fruit, lean protein, and whole grains can help you stay strong from start to finish. If you're exercising less than an hour, water is all you usually need to drink. If you are exercising for more than an hour (or in a hot and humid environment), have a sports drink containing glucose (sugar) and electrolytes (sodium, potassium, chloride, magnesium, calcium, etc.) on hand to keep you workout-ready. Sip as you exercise to stay energized and hydrated.

Dress the part.   Wearing the wrong shoes or clothing for a workout can make you uncomfortable and set you up for injury. Choose comfortable and appropriate fitting clothing and footwear for each type of exercise. If you're worried your sneakers may be worn out, buy new ones so you can get the support you need. It may sound silly, but I always recommend that fitness newbies do a dress rehearsal for their workouts to make sure their gym bags have all the right gear and their workout outfits fit right and provide the right blend of stretch and support. Nothing shuts down good exercise intentions faster than socks that bunch up when you walk or shoes that rub the wrong way. The type (mode) of fitness will determine the appropriate clothing and footwear needed. For example, the fitness session may require a bathing suit, cycling or running clothes, yoga or weight training clothes, layered clothing for outdoors, and a change of clothes. Be prepared for changing conditions, and bring a stopwatch to stay on time. What you wear does make a difference.

THE GOAL OF RESISTANCE

In The PRISE Life Protocol, the resistance routines are focused on developing muscular strength, power, and even endurance. There are hundreds of ways to get in your resistance training or strength training. You could use the leg press machine at your gym, do biceps curls with the use of a resistance band at your house, or even hold a plank position in your office. You can use weights or props to provide resistance and challenge your muscles, or you can stick to moves that use your own body weight, such as squats, lunges, pull-ups, or push-ups. In other words, there's no excuse not to integrate resistance workouts into your routine.

So, your workouts will focus on building lean muscle mass by using a combination of the following:

- Traditional weights (dumbbells, barbells, fitness equipment).
- Your body's own weight as resistance.
- Small props, such as an exercise band/tube, medicine ball, or kettlebell.

You'll work the large muscles first, overloading them, before focusing on your smaller muscles. This type of resistance training zaps total body and belly fat, increases lean muscle mass, and improves cardiovascular and metabolic health as well as enhances your mood.

The muscle mass you could gain from this type of exercise is impressive. In my PRISE study, some participants packed on close to eight pounds of lean body mass in twelve weeks! That's over a half-pound of muscle a week—the type of strength gains you can quickly see and feel. One woman I worked with went from being able to do just nine push-ups to mastering over twenty-five at a time; another was able to bench press an extra twenty-five pounds. All this from less than two months of working out!

Women, don't worry; you won't walk out looking like the Incredible Hulk, but it will define your muscles, especially your upper body, and that visceral fat (bad fat on your belly) and hip fat will start to disappear! When you perform the resistance training routine, aim to keep your intensity level between 7 and 10. Plus, the more muscle you have the more your body will burn off fat even while you are not working out. That's a huge benefit to increasing muscle mass.

My scientific research and experience with clients and athletes show this type of training reduces total body and belly fat, increases lean muscle mass, and improves cardiovascular, metabolic, and mood health. By building more muscle, as you do when you work the larger muscles like the glutes and quadriceps, you burn more calories, lose body fat, lower blood pressure, and increase your overall strength. Even if you're mostly interested in building strength and creating a more toned physique, you'll automatically get these other benefits too.

RESISTANCE TRAINING 101

Resistance exercise includes any physical movement that requires muscles to exert a force against some sort of resistance, whether it's gravity or a dumbbell. This force against resistance causes the muscle cells, sometimes referred to as fibers, to contract and change length. Resistance comes in three separate forms: concentric, eccentric and plyometric.

Most resistance exercises result in the shortening of muscle cells. These are *concentric* muscle contractions, such as a bicep curl. However, some resistance exercises cause muscle cells to lengthen. These are known as *eccentric* muscle contractions and include movements such as lowering a heavyweight to the floor. Lastly, a major component of resistance training is a form of muscle contraction called *plyometrics*. These are exercises that require the muscles to be rapidly stretched, and then immediately contracted, such as jumping off of a box onto the ground and then jumping onto another box (box jumping), or performing push-ups with a clap between them. The goal of plyometrics is to improve muscle power.

Whichever way the muscles are working (shortening or lengthening), they respond favorably to resistance training by improving the blood supply and nerve-conduction pathways to our muscles. It's sort of like construction work on a highway that adds another lane to make room for more vehicles and allows for easier transportation. The result is a more efficient transportation system to increase the speed in which oxygen and nutrients are delivered to help muscles repair damage and rebuild new muscle. Just as important, chronic resistance exercise training may help remove waste and release toxins that build up in muscles. The enhanced nerve pathways lead to smoother and faster-firing muscles, which is a very good thing. Taken together, the improved blood and nerve supply results in leaner muscles and better functioning and performing muscles.

The bones and joints also respond favorably to resistance exercise. Most people feel healthier, stronger, more fit, and better able to accomplish tasks and activities of daily living like climbing stairs or lifting heavy objects when they resistance train. You may find that your bone density scans improve when you start lifting weights and that your joints feel less achy thanks to the extra support your muscles are providing. I'm never surprised when I hear a test subject with arthritis in her knees say she's feeling a lot better after regularly doing lunges and squats.

For athletes, the increase in muscle function results in improved explosive power, strength, and agility, which translates to improved athletic performance. Runners and cyclists who add strength training to their routines are able to move faster for longer periods of time. Athletes may be able to jump higher or throw harder. Strengthening your muscles may allow you to lift heavier weights, but it'll also allow you to move better in all the things you do.

Circle the Exercises Performed from Each Category		Reps/ Time	Intensity
Dynamic Warm-up (Appendix C)	**Perform prior to each workout (Choose 7; 1 set; 7 minutes):** 1. Pendulum swings (side to side) 2. Pendulum swings (front to back) 3. High knee (chest) 4. High knee (external rotation) 5. Side shuffle 6. Carioca 7. Over-under the fence 8. Hip opening/closing 9. High knees 10. Butt kicks 11. Lunge with twist 12. Arm windmills		

Circle the Exercises Performed from Each Category	Reps/ Time	Intensity
Footwork And Agility	**Perform using agility ladder (Choose 4; 1 set; 4 minutes):** 1. Forward, double-step 2. Sideways, double-step 3. Side-step, double in/out 4. Side shuffle, two-in/out 5. Two-leg hops 6. One-leg hops 7. Two-leg hops, in/out 8. One-leg hops, in/out 9. One-leg hops, sideways 10. Side shuffle 11. Figure 8s 12. Kangaroo hops 2/1 foot 13. Kangaroo hops, sideways 14. T-drill 15. Jump rope		

Circle the Exercises Performed from Each Category	Reps/ Time	Intensity

Resistance AndPower Exercises	**Perform 6 below (2 sets; 12 minutes):**
	1. Side-steps toes in/out, ankles/ knees
	  - Side-steps with bands and med ball
	2. Forward/backward walk with bands
	3. Squats
	4. Lunges with tubing (with med ball)
	5. Lateral lunges (with med ball)
	6. Front step-ups
	7. Squat thrusts, med ball throws
	8. Jump squats
	9. Mountain climbers
	10. Squat-plank-jump squats
	11. Lateral step-ups
	Perform 6 below (2 sets; 12 minutes):
	1. Back rows/fly
	2. Pull-ups
	3. Chest press/fly
	4. Push-ups (choose one):
	  - side walking
	  - knees/toes w/physioball
	  - down dog
	  - side to side (ball)
	  - heart-to-heart
	  - hi/low
	5. Front/Lateral raises
	6. Biceps curls
	7. Shoulder press
	8. Hyperextensions		

Circle the Exercises Performed from Each Category	Reps/ Time	Intensity
Core Exercises	Perform 5 below (2 sets; 10 minutes): 1. Plank knees elbows/hands 2. Plank toes elbows/hands 3. Plank one leg elbows 4. Plank one leg hands on ball 5. Side planks foot-elbow/twist 6. Side planks hand stars 7. Airplanes 8. Superwoman/man 9. Crunches on ball 10. Plank with ball on knees/toes Perform 5 below (1 set; 5 minutes): 1. Knees to chest 2. Hyperextension on ball 3. Reverse planks one, two legs 4. Ab hollow		

*Cool down five minutes following R routine with gentle stretching. Total R exercise time is ~50–60 minutes.

BUILDING ON YOUR PRISE RESISTANCE TRAINING PLAN

PRISE contains an expansive and continuously growing number of resistance training options, and I've included the majority of them in my PRISE Life App (Apple App Store and Android Play Store). Remember, the resistance exercise training program is a series of exercises that incorporate dynamic, functional resistance movements of footwork/agility drills; bodyweight exercises involving weighted medicine balls, physioballs, exercise tubes and bands; and core-strengthening exercises.

Perform each exercise with enough weight or intensity (Intensity Level 7–10 using my scale) that your muscles are fatigued after either 30–40 seconds or 10 to 20 repetitions per set. You can change how hard you're working by lifting a heavier weight, using a thicker resistance band or tube, a heavier medicine ball, or moving more slowly or quickly.

Resistance exercises are absolutely wonderful and essential to getting stronger, healthier, and increasing your physical performance. The beauty is they don't have to be limiting. Don't forget that exercise can be done in places other than the gym. I designed it so you can perform these routines anywhere, anytime. One thing to keep in mind is that doing anything is usually better than nothing when it comes to general physical activity.

DAILY FITNESS HACKS FROM DR. PAUL

There are many small ways you can create a more active lifestyle without even trying. Here are some tips I recommend:

- Park at the farthest destination from your office, store or event.
- Leave your lunch in the car when you arrive at your office and then walk back out and get it.
- Every hour, walk to a coworker in another building or on a different floor or take a walk through the parking lot.
- When reading, watching TV or doing desk work at home or at work, make a point to stand up for 10-15 minutes every hour and stretch.
- Carry shopping/grocery bags versus using a cart.
- Practice diaphragmatic breathing (belly breathing) whenever you're feeling stressed.
- When waiting in line or at the airport, do some simple stretches.
- Any moment you have a chance to cherish nature, get outside or just breathe.

Don't take yourself too seriously in the beginning by comparing yourself to others at the gym. You are there for you, and soon you will be so thrilled you may be helping others!

And never, ever forget to have some fun! Bop in the pool, add a little tango to your warm-up, jive to some music, rap to some pumps, and by all means, remember that fitness was meant to be enjoyed, not torture!

Pretending you are Andre Agassi, one of the Williams sisters, Wayne Gretzky, an Olympian, or whatever gets your mind to help you move, is not only allowed, but encouraged. Your body, in its perfection, will have those endorphins pumping in no time, and you will finally start to enjoy it, "RISE Up," and actually want to do more of this exercise thing! No more excuses!

So, when you are smiling to yourself in the gym or accidentally grunting like Serena or Nadal, smile at yourself with pride or turn to your partner and say, "Dr. Paul told me to RISE Up!" That will be our little secret. But how you lost the fat and gained that muscle is something you can shout out to the world, especially as people start to ask you what you are doing to look so good. And remember, I'm constantly conducting new research studies on the effects of my PRISE Life Protocol using the best nutritional support available to maximize your results. So visit my website often to see what's coming up next (www.priselife.com).

CHAPTER 5
(I) IS FOR INTERVALS

Dr. Paul says: "Intervals help you sprint through life and relish the afterburn!"

PROTEIN PACING | RESISTANCE | **INTERVALS** | STRETCHING | ENDURANCE

"Slow and steady wins the race" is an often repeated saying that reminds us to slow down and take our time. This, of course, comes from the famous Aesop's fable of the tortoise and hare in which the overconfident, speedy rabbit challenges the turtle to a race and, despite sprinting away at the starting line, ends up falling asleep and losing to the slow-moving turtle. One takeaway from the story is that it doesn't pay to sprint through life. This chapter is short and sweet. If you understand interval training you'll be ahead of most people you may see working out in the gym. If you incorporate these suggestions into your PRISE Life routine, you'll be amazed at how effective they are. Intervals are one of the lesser-known keys to overall fitness and will help you see steady and consistent results. And like the quote above, an added side effect of intervals is that some previously closed roads in your life may begin to fly open for you.

WHAT IS INTERVAL TRAINING?

When it comes to your health and fitness, "sprinting" in the form of high-intensity interval exercise is one of the most effective ways to burn fat, build muscle, strengthen the heart, and increase metabolism. Intervals are simply the staggering of slow and fast segments of cardio during the course of your workout. Research shows that alternating slow and fast segments of cardio is one of the best ways to improve your health.

To do an interval, you're going to walk, jog, swim, row, or cycle super fast, then slow down enough to recover and catch your breath. This sort of exercise improves cardiovascular fitness, increases lean muscle mass and metabolism, and reduces body fat, belly fat, and blood sugar. Plus, it's quick! With intervals, you can exercise for less than thirty minutes, yet you'll be stronger and feel more energized when you finish. This is a good way to gain fitness fast. With intervals, some of my PRISE testers improved their cardiovascular fitness by more than 80% in eight weeks. That means no more huffing and puffing up the stairs!

Interval training is often shown using a ratio of exercise to recovery. For example, you might do one minute of work, then recover for two minutes. It's these changes in intensity that make a workout an interval workout. You work hard and fast, and when you're about to tucker out you take a short break—usually to catch your breath—then you do it all again.

And please don't be fooled into thinking that intervals are only for the top athletes. Research consistently shows that intervals are one of the most effective and safest training strategies for the obese, type 2 diabetics, and cardiac rehabilitation patients! In other words, intervals are great for everyone, no matter your fitness or health status or age or gender. So let's start sprinting together.

The people I work with love intervals because they are time-efficient. You can exercise for less than thirty minutes and you'll feel stronger and more energized when you finish. Interval training can be applied to just about any type of aerobic activity, including walking, jogging, swimming, or cycling. If you can speed it up or slow it down, you can add intervals.

INTERVAL TRAINING SPEEDS UP RESULTS

Most people think the best way to lose body fat, especially belly fat, is through endurance or aerobic exercise; the opposite is actually true. A growing body of scientific evidence shows that interval training is the best way to enhance aerobic fitness and turn your body into a fat-burning machine! Not only do intervals add excitement to your usual cardio routines, but they are a much more time-efficient way to fitness and leanness.

So instead of heading out for a steady run or bike ride, carefully monitor your time, going hard or easing up based on how you feel using my intensity scale and by what your watch says in terms of the time or heart rate. Your brain will be busy, and your body will be working in a new and challenging way. But this isn't some simple diversion tactic. Intervals really do make your workout effective. Research shows that staggering slow and fast segments of cardio is one of the best ways to improve cardiovascular fitness, increase lean muscle mass and metabolism, and reduce body fat, belly fat, and blood sugar.

Interval training automatically improves fitness. Most people are aware that when you run at a steady state, such as when you set the treadmill to 6 mph, your body gets into a rhythm. This is perfect for endurance training—if you tap out at thirty minutes one day, you might be able to eke out thirty-two minutes the next, and so on. Your body gets a little bit stronger with each workout. What most don't realize is that this is true for intervals. You can increase your endurance in the same way, but you'll also be increasing your power and speed.

THE AFTERBURN OF AN INTERVAL WORKOUT

For example, say you're that person who regularly runs at 6 mph. What would happen if you were to bump up your speed to 8 or even 8.5 or 9 mph? You could probably keep up for a short period of time, such as thirty to sixty seconds. After that, you'd have to come back down to a very slow walk of 2.5 to 3 mph to catch your breath. That's how intervals work. You step outside of your comfort zone, building muscular endurance as well as speed and power.

Over time, if you practice this way it might take you less time to get to your top speed, and you will be able to sprint faster and faster as time goes on. I tend to recommend that people start training with a 1:3 interval ratio—one minute of all-out exercise for every three minutes of recovery. As your fitness levels improve, you might notice that you need a slightly longer time to recover because you are pushing yourself even harder during the sprint interval.

Part of what fuels this gain in speed, endurance, and power is a gain in muscle tone. When you really push yourself, you're bound to grow muscle fibers. As you already know, this increase in muscle leads to a boost in daily calorie burn. For each pound you add, you can expect to burn about an extra hundred calories a day. However, that's just one way intervals lead to a higher all-day calorie burn.

One of my favorite aspects of intervals—and one you're going to love too—is a change in several key enzymes inside our muscle cells that create the "afterburn." In science-speak, afterburn means the period of time you continue to burn energy (or calories) after a workout. Although you may be done exercising, your body is still in a high metabolic state, which means you're zapping extra calories automatically. Imagine that you sit for an hour and, in doing so, burn sixty calories. Then you do an intense interval workout for thirty minutes, revving your heart rate, breathing, body temperature, hormone levels, and metabolism. For up to seventy-two hours after you exercise, you'll be burning more calories than before. You may sit back down after your workout and burn 120 calories in that first hour, and one hundred calories in the second hour. Tack that on to the calories you burn during the actual workout, and you can start to see why intervals are so good for weight and fat loss.

THE INTERVAL WORKOUT

Intervals are part work, part recovery. When you're starting out, your recovery time is going to be a lot longer than your periods of work. You may sprint for one minute, then gently jog for two or three minutes. As you improve, your work periods may get a little shorter, and your rest periods may get a little longer because you learn to push yourself harder. The more conditioned you are, the easier it will be for you to catch your breath, feel your heart rate come back down, and feel prepared to give it your all again.

You can customize your own sprint-and-recover routine or choose one option from below.

Option 1: Thirty-second intervals at Level 10 (Sprint Interval Training, SIT)	Perform a thirty-second sprint interval at an "all-out" intensity (Intensity Level 10), followed by a four-minute recovery at Intensity Level 2. Repeat seven times. NOTE: This would be written as 7 X 30 seconds: Four minutes, indicating seven sets of "all-out" exercise for thirty seconds, followed by a four-minute recovery.

Option 2: Sixty-second intervals at Level 9 (High-Intensity Interval Training, HIIT)	Perform a sixty-second sprint interval at an almost all-out intensity (Intensity Level 9), followed by a two-minute recovery at Intensity Level 2. Repeat nine times. NOTE: This would be written as 9 X 60 seconds: Two minutes, indicating nine sets of almost all-out exercise for sixty seconds, followed by a two-minute recovery.

You will want to start and end each interval workout with a warm-up and a cool-down. At the beginning and end of each interval session, perform a five-minute dynamic warm-up. After you're done with the complete round of intervals, finish your workout with a gentle cool-down stretch session. (See the Resistance Training chapter for complete instructions on the dynamic warm-up and cool-down sections.) Each complete interval workout will take between thirty and forty minutes.

When broken down by time, this is what Option 1 looks like:

0:00 to 5:00	Dynamic warm-up (see Resistance Training chapter for complete instructions)
5:00 to 5:30	Sprint at Intensity Level 10
5:30 to 9:00	Recover at Intensity Level 2
9:00 to 9:30	Sprint at Intensity Level 10
9:30 to 13:30	Recover at Intensity Level 2
13:30 to 14:00	Sprint at Intensity Level 10
14:00 to 17:00	Recover at Intensity Level 2
17:00 to 17:30	Sprint at Intensity Level 10
17:30 to 21:00	Recover at Intensity Level 2
21:00 to 21:30	Sprint at Intensity Level 10
21:30 to 25:00	Recover at Intensity Level 2
25:00 to 25:30	Sprint at Intensity Level 10
25:30 to 29:30	Recover at Intensity Level 2

29:30 to 30:00	Sprint at Intensity Level 10
30:00 to 32:00	Recover at Intensity Level 2
32:00 to 35:00	Gentle cool-down

Here is a chart of the interval workout options:

Interval Training (I) — Option 1

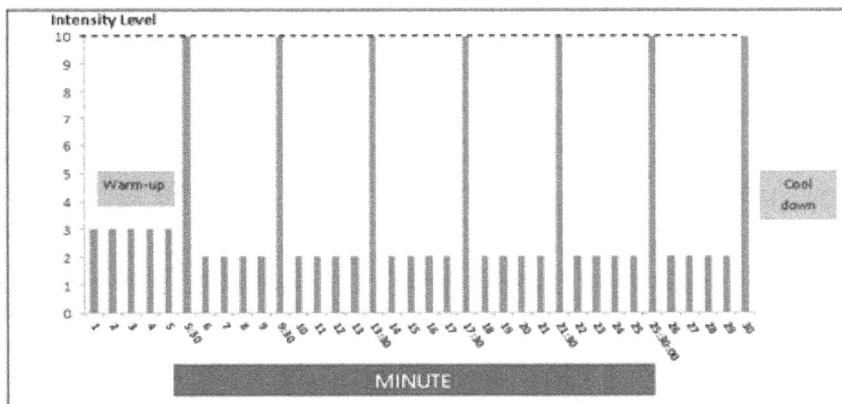

Interval Training (I) — Option 2

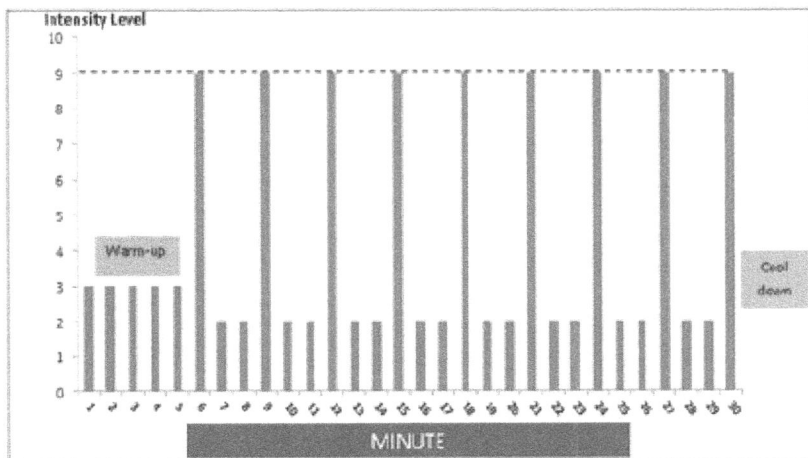

DR. PAUL'S CAUTION ABOUT INTERVALS

Intervals are an intense exercise routine, so be careful not to overdo it. Allow at least four days between interval sessions, and I recommend you perform each RISE routine one day per week for a total of four days of exercise per week. After the first four weeks, feel free to choose one of the RISE routines to perform a second time, but I recommend not to exceed five days of exercise per week because your body needs time to recover, replenish, and rebuild.

Always perform the dynamic warm-up before and a gentle cool-down after each session. Remember, this is always about work, then recovery. However, the great news is that recovery has new meaning because just think, with the "afterburn" working for you—instead of against you, when you go to relax—you will be burning more calories, even up to as long as seventy-two hours, than you would have if you had not done your interval training. That's motivation right there!

As stated above, this exercise routine has been scientifically proven to strengthen your heart, burn body fat, build muscle, and increase your metabolic rate (burn more calories), leading to improved overall health. It is also one of the most time-efficient forms of exercise you can perform. I know things are so hectic these days that many of us are sprinting through life, but that is not the long-term answer. By doing these targeted sprints and resting when needed, we will win the race of a long, healthy, vital, and productive life.

CHAPTER 6
(S) IS FOR STRETCHING

Dr. Paul says: "Stretching is the
glue that holds the body together."

PROTEIN PACING | RESISTANCE | INTERVALS | **STRETCHING** | ENDURANCE

During a recent television interview in which I discussed health and wellness, one of the producers asked me what I thought about stretching and yoga exercises. Interestingly, this is the most common exercise and fitness question I am asked, and my reply is always the same: Stretching, flexibility, and yoga are the glue that holds the body together, and in their absence, your body would fall apart and your risk of injury would increase dramatically.

Our muscular and skeletal systems function like pulleys and levers; therefore, they need to be kept well-lubricated and aligned properly. In addition, our tendons and muscles, which function like the cables of the pulley, need to be adequately stretched and cared for to prevent them from becoming stiff and brittle and even tearing. Stretching exercises are particularly important the more physically active we are and especially as we age. A regular stretching and flexibility routine that moves the joints, tendons, ligaments, and muscles through a range of motion is critical to maintaining optimal health and function. This type of exercise routine may take different forms, such as simple stretching, yoga, qigong, Tai Chi, and Pilates, but the important point is, it needs to be done consistently on a weekly basis.

Stretching can be done in a lot of different ways, but my favorite is yoga. I trained to get my yoga teaching certifications a few years ago because it seemed like the perfect complement to the more intense types of exercise I do. Stretching and practicing yoga poses, or asanas, can increase flexibility, balance, and muscle tone and give you a greater sense of tranquility and peacefulness. Stretching is also restorative because it improves balance, muscle tone, and flexibility, but it can also lower blood sugar and even enhance mood. Having trouble touching your toes? Not for long! In this program, exercisers saw their hamstring flexibility improve by more than four inches, and they felt a lot more relaxed in stressful situations. Who doesn't want that?

TWO TYPES OF STRETCHING

When you stretch, you may feel a small tug in your muscles. Or you might simply feel your joints warming and opening. Both of these results are likely the byproduct of dynamic stretching and static stretching, the main types of stretching/flexibility exercises you need to follow:

1) Dynamic (best done during a warm-up)
2) Static (best done during a cool-down)

Dynamic stretches are active movements such as swinging, sweeping, twisting, and stepping. Dynamic stretching means moving through various ranges of motion, not just holding one position. These are often used as warm-up exercises.

Dynamic stretching will enhance physical performance and muscle action as well as reduce injury because it prepares the muscles for movement by activating the nerves and muscle fibers. Warming up the muscles prior to stretching or movement increases the delivery of vital oxygen and nutrients to the muscles, which are necessary to provide movement. (Cue up the image of pro athletes getting warmed up before a big game.) Dynamic stretches are active in nature. You move continuously through a full range of motion in an attempt to "wake up" or activate your muscles, tendons, ligaments, and bones so you are absolutely ready to perform whatever sport or activity you're preparing for.

Static stretches are your quintessential stretches. You find a position that tests your flexibility, and then you hold it. This type of stretching usually involves holding a specific stretch for ten seconds or longer. Static stretching should be done only when the muscles are warm and there is increased blood flow and circulation. This will enhance recovery from intense exercise training as well as reduce injury because it properly stretches the muscles and helps enhance blood flow and the removal of waste products.

Static stretching is best performed as a confined "Stretching" exercise routine or after you've performed resistance, interval or endurance exercise. You may have heard that you should reserve five to ten minutes for static stretching after you have exercised. That's the perfect time to do it, since your muscles will be plenty warm, and stretching can improve your recovery from the hard work. However, you can also perform this type of stretching during workouts such as yoga, Pilates, and Tai Chi.

STRETCHING IMPROVES YOUR BODY'S BALANCE

Who has time for stretching? I get it. All you want to do is move, to feel like you're really shedding pounds, zapping calories, and building strength. But integrating stretching or stretch-based workouts such as yoga will benefit your other workouts.

Stretching helps with at least five types of physical and emotional balance to the body.

1) It can add length to muscles that are getting stronger and shorter. This is important because most athletes benefit from a large range of motion. (There are, of course, some exceptions where tight muscles can help your performance, but unless you're an Olympic hopeful, you probably don't need to worry about this.)

2) Stretching can also address imbalances in the body, creating symmetry, stability, and better form. If a swimmer has one flexible shoulder and one tight one, they aren't going to cover the length of the pool as quickly or easily if their range of motion was equal.

3) The toned-down energy required during stretching or yoga is a good counter to workouts such as resistance and intervals. You're moving some—enough to relieve delayed onset muscle soreness and increase your circulation—but not enough to tire you out. In fact, you might even feel like you're taking a recovery day, which is a must for proper maintenance.

4) Stretching—at least in the form of yoga poses—can improve your balance as you learn to hold precarious poses without wobbling or wiggling.

5) But my favorite reason to practice stretching exercises and yoga poses is that it naturally increases mood and lowers anxiety by elevating brain levels of the neurotransmitter gamma-aminobutyric acid (GABA). This finding alone should have you running out to buy a yoga mat and then get started with my PRISE stretching routine! Most conventional pharmacological medications/drugs prescribed with the goal of improving mood and lowering anxiety aim to increase GABA levels, but usually are accompanied by side effects. Stretching and yoga may provide the same benefits but without the side effects.

As with everything else I suggest in this book, I practice what I preach. As a certified yoga instructor in two different forms, I've led thousands of people through yoga workouts—from CEOs to top athletes to everyday people who want to feel more fit and enjoy a healthier lifestyle. I also regularly do my own yoga workouts. I've found it's the best way for me to enhance my muscle flexibility and joint mobility and at the same time reconnect my mind to my body.

My favorite time to do my Stretching routine is after a strenuous Resistance, Interval or Endurance workout the day before. In this plan, you only need to do one sixty-minute stretching workout each week. But if you find you like to do more—waking up with five minutes of yoga or fitting in a few stretching poses in the afternoon—I encourage you to do so. Unlike the other type of training in the RISE program, it's quite hard to overdo stretching. The type of stretching you do is less important than the regularity with which you do it. For stretching to be effective, you must do it on a regular weekly basis.

THE WORKOUT

The stretching routine in this program involves traditional yoga poses called "asanas," with a combination of core and strengthening elements for a total body workout that will leave you rejuvenated and recharged. You can always follow along in The PRISE Life app, which you've hopefully downloaded already.

Warm-Up Stretches:

- Warm-up Stretches (Sun Salutations):
- Mountain Pose (Tadasana)
- Standing Forward Bend (Uttanasana)
- Plank Pose (Phalakasana)

- Four-Limbed Staff Pose (Chaturanga Dandasana)
- Cobra Pose (Bhujangasana)
- Upward Facing Dog Pose (Urdhva Mukha Svanasana)
- Downward Facing Dog Pose (Adha Mukha Svanasana)
- Child's Pose/Rest Pose (Balasana)

Standing Stretches:

- Neck Stretching
- Side Bending
- Lunge Pose (Anjaneyasana)
- Warrior I Pose (Virabhadrasana I)
- Warrior II Pose (Virabhadrasana II)
- Triangle Pose (Utthita Trikonasana)
- Extended Side Angle Pose (Utthita Parsvakonasana)
- Goddess Pose (Utkata Konasana)
- Chair Pose (Utkatasana)
- Revolved Chair Pose (Parivrtta Utkatasana)
- Squat Pose (Malasana)
- Standing Wide-Legged Forward Bend Pose (Prasarita Padottanasana)

Balance in Motion Stretches:

- Tree Pose (Vrksasana)
- Warrior III (Virabhadrasana III)
- Lord of the Dance Pose (Natarajasana)
- Standing One-Legged Balance
- Eagle Pose (Garudasana)
- Boat Pose (Navasana)
- Bicycle Pose
- Bow Pose (Dhanurasana)
- Candlestick Pose

- Camel Pose (Ustrasana)
- Pigeon Pose (Eke Pada Rajakapotasana)

Floor Stretches:

- Seated Cross-Legged Pose (Sukhasana)
- Staff Pose (Dandasana)
- eated Forward Bend (Paschimottanasana)
- Head to Knee Pose (Janu Sirsasana)
- Wide Seated Forward Bend Pose (Upavistha Konasana)
- Table Top Pose and Cat/Cow
- Bridge Pose (Setu Bandhasana)
- Extended Puppy Dog Pose (Uttana Shishosana)
- Butterfly Pose (Baddha Konasana)
- Happy Baby Pose (Ananda Balasana)
- Half Twist Pose (Ardha Matsyendrasana)
- Head to Knee Pose (Janu Sirsasana)
- Front Split Pose (Hanumanasana)
- Frog Pose (Mandukasana)
- Spinal Twist Pose (Supta Matsyendrasana)
- Corpse Pose (Savasana)
- Reclining Bound Angle Pose (Supta Baddha Konasana)

If you stretch in a gentle but regular way, you'll gradually open up your muscles, making it easier to exercise and also increase your ability to do everyday things, like reaching for items on the top shelf or picking things off the floor and maintaining your balance on uneven or slippery surfaces. Of course, if you don't take stretching seriously or don't try to push yourself a little more each time you reach for your toes or open your arms wide, you won't see many changes.

On the other hand, if you push yourself away into the uncomfortable zone, you may be able to touch your toes, but you may get there by tearing your hamstring or otherwise injuring yourself. To find that middle ground, I encourage people to bring the stretch to the "soft edge," that place where you feel the tightness in the muscle but bring your awareness and your breath to the tightness and then breathe past it. This is a really cool place to be because it heightens your awareness and mindfulness of your body. In a short time, you may be enjoying yourself so much that you'll want to commit more than one day a week to it!

Stretching creates flexibility, pliability, and mobility, and these create strength and power and keep you injury-free. The amazing thing is that this is not only true of our muscles, but also of our emotions and mindset. People who can't face change or who are inflexible cause themselves to suffer in more ways than necessary. They create energy around them that makes it difficult to grow or to find deep peace and understanding of others.

Every day is such a gift that if we allow our minds to grow, to be flexible, if we work it like our muscles, if we stretch ourselves and our beliefs, we will discover that the world and people have so much more to offer. It is why the great masters who have lived and taught us through the centuries have had so many answers to the baffling questions we struggle with about the universe. When you think about what Liezi teaches when he says, "Develop flexibility and you will be firm; cultivate yielding and you will be strong," understand that this goes much deeper than the muscles themselves. In Chapter 12, we'll go more in-depth about the practice of integrative health and the importance of turning inward to master the world around us.

CHAPTER 7
(E) IS FOR ENDURANCE

Dr. Paul says: "Endurance is nature's aphrodisiac."

PROTEIN PACING | RESISTANCE | INTERVALS | STRETCHING | **ENDURANCE**

Yes, diamonds are proof of endurance, as they often take between one and three billion years to form! Don't worry, I'm not asking that much of you, and whether we agree with the Forbes fortune or not, diamonds definitely stick to their jobs and demonstrate the ultimate endurance. In the fitness world, endurance is another name for cardiovascular or aerobic exercise—those long and continuous jogs, walks, swims, or bike rides. Doing this kind of exercise for an hour or more is one of the surest ways to help lower blood pressure and blood sugar, both of which reduce your risk for heart disease and type 2 diabetes. This type of exercise also includes running, swimming, hiking, cross-country skiing, snowshoeing, rollerblading, and rowing, among other sports.

Endurance exercise is good for your body, and it also has a tremendous effect on brain health, including enhanced cognition, brain function, and feelings of happiness. It can also help reduce feelings of depression, tension, and anxiety. People talk about the "runner's high," but it can really come from any type of continuous endurance activity.

RESEARCH ON ENDORPHINS

Several years ago, I read a fascinating research study from Germany that documented the runner's high in humans for the first time. By definition, the runner's high is an enhanced mood state that occurs during or following endurance exercise of more than an hour.

It's related to a flood of endorphins in the brain. Endorphins are chemicals released by the body during a handful of activities, including extreme or thrill-seeking sports like skydiving, rock climbing, heli-skiing, endurance exercise, laughter, and sex. They're often called "feel-good chemicals," since they block feelings of stress or pain. Endorphins are associated with feelings of euphoria, happiness, and even extreme peacefulness. The more endorphins that are released during exercise, the more intense the feelings.

Until this study, the runner's high was mostly anecdotal and had never been proven to exist from a scientific standpoint. However, the findings provided first-hand evidence that exercise ($\geq$ 60 minutes) increases endorphin release in the brain as well as feelings of euphoria and happiness.

As an avid endurance athlete myself, I have experienced the runner's high for decades, so this study validated that my feelings were not imagined. More importantly, the study proved that the runner's high is real, and performing endurance exercise increases feelings of euphoria, happiness, and peacefulness—it's the purest form of a natural high. Endurance exercise can be addictive because of the runner's high.

THE HEALTHY SIDE EFFECTS OF ENDURANCE

One of my favorite side effects of endurance exercise is the opportunity to experience synchrony among all the different systems of the body, such as the beating of my heart, the rhythm of my breathing, and the contraction of my muscles—often referred to as entrainment. This occurs most commonly when you are performing endurance exercise and using your full body in a rhythmical movement pattern, such as jogging/running, cycling, or swimming, and your breathing, heartbeat, and muscle contractions all begin to work in synchrony. It's a beautiful occurrence when it happens, and I've experienced it often during my days as an endurance/triathlete. It's like a symphony, with all the moving parts working together to create something much bigger than the individual parts.

This is what happens when we perform endurance training using entrainment. The heartbeat, lungs, muscles, and nervous system are each capable of supporting the exercise independently of each other; however, when they are working synchronously, the result is magnificent—exercise becomes almost effortless, tremendously enjoyable, almost meditative and spiritual in nature.

This is the goal of the Endurance exercise routine, to become transformative and to bring you to another dimension of self-awareness/actualization. I like to perform the endurance routine out in nature and first thing in the morning because it's so serene, peaceful, and quiet and the body is still relatively silent. And at 60%–70% intensity, it results in the greatest brain blood flow and most likely setting for a euphoric runner's high and mood boost!

If you're intimidated by the idea of endurance activity—or exercising continuously for an hour or more—let that feeling go. All of you reading this are capable of performing an endurance routine using the guidelines I provide. Indeed, you probably already do some sort of endurance training, whether it's in the form of walking up and down the aisles of the grocery store, playing in a recreational soccer game, heading out on an afternoon hike, or swimming some laps. All continuous activity counts, even if it's gentle movement. Of course, for the maximum benefits, the intensity needs to be such that you're at least a little breathless.

ENDURANCE 101

Endurance exercise includes any type of activity that engages the majority of your body mass. This includes walking, jogging, running, cycling, swimming, hiking, cross-country skiing, snowshoeing, rollerblading, rowing, and dancing. Of course, you can do all of these activities as intervals or as short workouts. To make sure you're training to effectively increase your endurance, you must keep going for an hour or longer.

What's so important about sixty minutes (or more) of activity? By exercising for this amount of time, you begin to illuminate receptors in your brain that are associated with feelings of euphoria and happiness, which ultimately leads to the natural high people experience while engaged in endurance exercise. This is much more likely to happen while we are in the naturalistic environment of the outdoors in nature.

With endurance work, the formula is still the same. You're going to schedule a sixty-minute or longer endurance exercise session each week. Even if you're an absolute beginner, you can keep going for a full hour. Just focus on starting slow and slightly increasing your speed each time. You may start walking and build up to simply walking with more intensity, something you can accomplish by increasing your speed, finding a place to walk that has a slight incline so you're walking uphill, and even by pumping your arms more vigorously. Remember, only achieve a Level 6 on my Intensity scale.

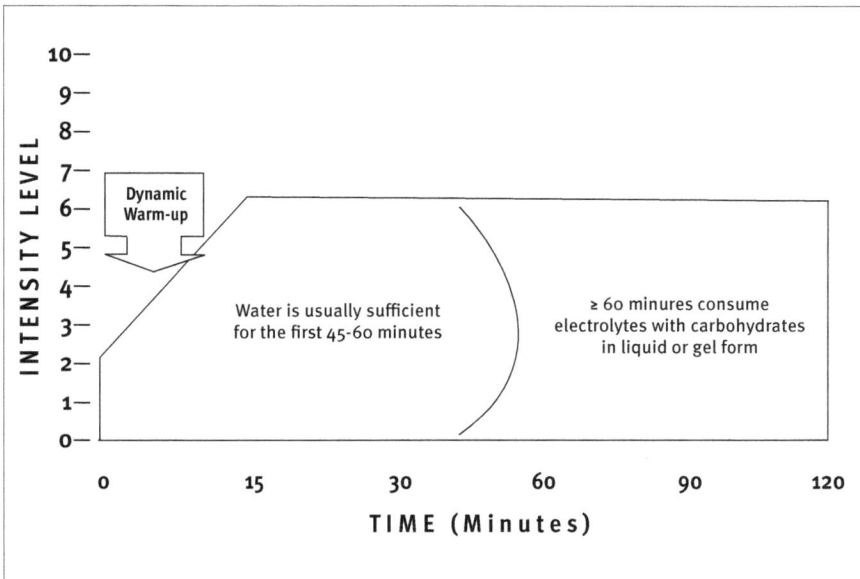

THE BENEFITS OF AN OUTDOOR WORKOUT

Those who know me know that I am a huge proponent of performing most physical exercise outdoors in nature, so you can truly disconnect from your wired world and connect to your inner world. By your inner world, I am, of course, referring to the harmony of you: spirit, mind, and body.

While I fully understand, appreciate, and have even proven through scientific research that performing the exercise while virtually engaged with an interactive video game (called exergaming) is beneficial for our brain health in certain circumstances, I also believe that exercising outdoors has superior health benefits compared to indoor exercise.

The best news is there is now scientific evidence to support my belief.

Researchers from the Peninsula College of Medicine and Dentistry in the UK analyzed data from 833 adults and showed that their mental well-being was improved while exercising outdoors compared to exercising indoors. Hence, the name "nature pill." Some of the health benefits included increased energy, feelings of engagement, joy, and satisfaction, along with decreased tension, confusion, anger, and depression.

Use any mode of exercise that incorporates the majority of your body (swimming, walking, running, cycling, cross-country skiing, rollerblading, skating, snow shoeing, hiking, etc.). At the beginning of each endurance session, remember to perform that five- minute dynamic warm-up and a gentle stretch when you finish.

While I have consistently urged people to perform endurance exercise outdoors as a way to enjoy themselves, it is also a way to dramatically improve their psychological well being. Fortunately, these current research findings support my hunch. When you exercise outdoors, you will likely "think" and "feel" better, which may lead to making better lifestyle choices. Science says your stress level, as measured by the stress hormone cortisol, also plummets when you've engaged in a nature pill endurance bout.

Therefore, instead of only using endurance exercise to help burn more calories, focus on the improved mood state effects that may result and may lead to healthy lifestyle choices, such as choosing higher-quality foods to nourish your body. In fact, there is evidence that endurance exercise may promote food intake, making it harder to curb your appetite. By performing endurance exercise outdoors in nature, it may offset the increased food intake by enhancing your mood, leading to better food choices. Now that's fascinating!

MORE ENDURANCE WORKOUT BENEFITS

Endurance exercise is very beneficial for improving your body's ability to metabolize sugar in your blood and for lowering your blood pressure, two extremely important health benefits that drastically reduce your risk for heart disease and diabetes. The bottom line is that you need to adopt the understanding that performing endurance exercise in nature extends beyond the calories you burn while doing so. It also improves your overall mood state and reduces your risk for heart disease and diabetes. So get up from the couch and make an appointment with Mother Nature today!

It's wonderful to know that with this type of activity, aside from the pride of knowing your body is strong enough to go-go-go for an hour or more, you are helping protect your body from illness and premature aging. It's exciting to know it burns major calories and positively increases brain health, including enhanced cognition, brain function, and mood state.

In layman's terms, this means you might find you have an easier time remembering things, solving problems, and managing stress all day long! As a bonus, at the end of a long bout of endurance activity, you might get a huge burst of happiness—Mother Nature's aphrodisiac or runner's high. In this case, it's Dr. Paul approved!

A WORD ABOUT FITNESS/NUTRITION TRACKERS

"How many calories have you eaten today?" "How many steps have you taken today?" The modern world is so very different if you're one of the millions of people tracking every morsel of food you've eaten. In fact, you probably know how many calories you've burned too.

While we've covered Protein Pacing in detail and the RISE fitness program to complete our PRISE Life protocol, in the last few chapters, you may be wondering if a fitness tracker could be helpful. Here are my thoughts on that.

An eye-opening statistic stated that there were 90 million wearable nutrition, fitness, and health-monitoring devices sold in 2014, and it is projected that the market will grow from $4 billion in 2015 to over $40 billion in 2020! So what makes these nutrition, health, and fitness-tracking devices so popular? For most people, it's the awareness of eating an appropriate number of calories and staying active during the day, especially if you haven't met your "step" or "calorie" goal. To put it simply, they do a good job of motivating users to remain active and eat the appropriate number of calories.

And these devices attempt to do so much more. Some measure heart rate and variability, blood oxygen level, respiration rate, skin temperature, sweat rate, sleep patterns, etc., and soon they will be capturing vital personal biometrics, such as blood sugar, blood pressure, and blood lipids.

However, I do offer a word of caution. Because these self-monitoring devices are undergoing such rapid evolution, a major concern is their ongoing accuracy. Indeed, a recent article in *The Journal of the American Medical Association* highlights the variability of measurement (accuracy) among these different devices.

As a matter of interest, I've been publishing scientific research studies using data from these technologies and devices for over a decade, so they're not new to me. The ones I use for my scientific research studies have been validated and shown to be fairly accurate. I cannot say the same for the ones currently on the market. In any case, they were originally developed to provide an estimate, not a direct measure of the calories eaten and the calories burned during physical activity, so it's probably not a wise idea to create a balance sheet of the calories burned using these devices and the calories you are allowed to eat. This approach will leave you frustrated, because you'll be either starving or plump.

In my view, a major limitation of all the current self-monitoring technologies and tracking devices is their overzealous focus on measuring the quantity of each lifestyle metric. Their goal is a zero-sum game of measuring the *number* of steps and calories, monitoring sleep and heart rate, breath and beads of sweat, and there is little if any attention to the *quality* of these lifestyle experiences. *In support of this, countless well-respected scientists and studies have documented that the quality of our lifestyle choices is much more important than the quantity of each of these aspects of health.* And none is more scientifically proven than The PRISE Life Protocol.

For example, simply recommending more exercise as a public health initiative is considerably less effective than encouraging a balanced routine incorporating a variety of movement experiences such as resistance, interval, stretching, and endurance exercises as part of my PRISE Life Protocol. And I have the published research to back this up. Similarly, telling someone to simply "eat less" to lose weight is not very helpful, healthy, or motivating in the long term. Whereas providing help and guidance with choosing the right type of high-quality, nourishing foods, especially protein using my Protein Pacing plan, is paramount to effective, healthy weight loss and body composition.

Recently, I've been interviewed to comment on these nutrition and fitness technologies and tracking devices. I encourage you to watch it at www.priselife.com. My take-home message emphasizes the potential benefit these technologies will provide for workplace wellness to increase productivity, morale, and, most importantly, health. The cost savings will be enormous to employers, employees, and the entire workforce.

Herein lies the next phase of nutrition, health, and fitness technologies. The industry is primed to develop a combination nutrition/health app and fitness tracking device that emphasizes the quality of lifestyle choices above and beyond the quantified self.

Fortunately, I've been consulted by the health and wellness and health-care industries to provide a novel approach of personalized nutrition, fitness, and emotional well-being using my PRISE Life App. So go ahead and use a wearable tracker, but focus on the quality of your food and exercise over the quantity of calories and steps you take. Monitor but don't obsess. Follow The PRISE Life plan using my PRISE Life app and you'll be looking and feeling better in no time, with or without a tracker.

DR. PAUL'S PRISE TIPS FOR ENDURANCE

- **Aim for an Intensity Level of 6 out of 10.** What does Six feel like? This is a level of activity where you can have a conversation with a friend for hours. You may be breathing a little heavy, but you can still spit out full sentences and even paragraphs of dialogue.

- **Get out in nature.** Studies show that going out into the woods, a grassy field, or even a park for a "nature pill" can make you feel even happier and more revitalized. (Of course, if you fire up the treadmill on days when there's bad weather, you may feel even better being inside!)

- **Move first thing in the morning.** Just like the stretching workout, I'd recommend you do this right after getting out of bed, either before you have eaten (I call this "Fasted Endurance," others may refer to it as "Fasted Cardio") or after a small morning snack. Make sure you take a moment to first hydrate with water, tea, or a little morning java without cream and sugar.

- **Refuel as needed.** If you plan to exercise for more than sixty minutes, bring along extra nourishment, just in case. You might find you prefer a sports drink with electrolytes, a small packet of trail mix, or an energy gel. After one hour of moving, your body and brain may need this extra fuel to keep going strong.

- **Ditch the distractions**. You may want to scroll past this suggestion, but I would strongly recommend you exercise without any electronic devices, except maybe a watch or heart rate monitor. That means no music, no TV, no checking email. (For you old-schoolers, no paper books or magazines either!) This will allow you to tune in to your own body rhythms, feeling and listening to your body's feedback as you exercise. Noticing your breath, heart rate, and the general feeling of effort you're putting out can help you decide to speed up, slow down, or otherwise change your workout.

This is called being mindful and present with your body, and it is one surefire way to become a better athlete.

THE FINAL FRONTIER OF FASTED ENDURANCE

The Fasted Endurance (or fasted cardio) routine has really caught on recently, especially for those interested in losing weight and body fat. I've experimented with this myself and found it to be a mildly effective strategy to accelerate body fat loss if done properly. Specifically, Fasted Endurance is performed first thing in the morning following an overnight fast with nothing but water, coffee, or tea drank prior to exercising. The idea is that your body is in a low fuel (energy) state and primarily relying on fat as the major fuel source. If you go for a longer run, cycle, or swim first thing in the morning before you've eaten any food, your body will kick into a higher rate of fat burning to fuel the exercise you are doing. But it also has some major shortcomings that may jeopardize your weight- and fat-loss goals. Let me explain.

By the time you wake after a night's sleep of 7-8 hours, your body fuel/ energy stores of carbohydrates are nearly depleted, leaving you primarily your fat stores to be burned. Unfortunately, your body is also not synthesizing (building new) protein in this state. In fact, it is beginning to break down your body protein stores, including your muscle, as a potential energy source. So while you may be accelerating fat burning during Fasted Endurance/cardio, you are also breaking down and losing more protein from your muscles.

There is one other major setback I let people know about, which is that is your body is very smart and always on high alert when it senses you are going down a dangerous path, and will do whatever it can (adapt) to prevent injury. In the case of Fasted Endurance/cardio, the body will counteract the addition of exercise to a fasted state with a lowering or blunting of your metabolism to safeguard against an unsafe or unhealthy level of energy expenditure. In other words, your body's metabolism compensates by adjusting to a lower level of calorie burning during the exercise and over time may simply recalibrate to a lower metabolism all the time, making it even more difficult to burn calories and shed the weight and fat. As a result, I do not recommend Fasted Endurance/cardio on a regular basis. Instead, I advise my clients to do it no more than once per week and only up to four weeks at a time, and then take a break for at least four weeks.

Here are my recommendations and cautions of Fasted Endurance:

1) Aim for a maximum of sixty minutes per session at Intensity Level 6 or 7.

2) Perform no more than one time per week for no more than four weeks at a time.

3) Make sure to replenish, refuel, and rehydrate with electrolytes (sodium, potassium, magnesium, chloride, calcium) during and after, along with 20–40g of high-quality protein within two hours of finishing the workout.

It's super important to follow these guidelines for Fasted Endurance to maximize the fat-burning, maintain adequate hydration and muscle function, and minimize lean muscle mass loss and a lowering of metabolism (calorie burn at rest) that commonly occurs with repeated or inappropriate Fasted Endurance. I want to let you in on a little secret: "Fasted Core" is a much more effective fitness routine to shred abs and burn belly fat than Fasted Endurance. I explain this in-depth in The PRISE Life Playbook.

CONCLUSION

I want to conclude this section of the book by sharing how excited I am that you are now equipped with the knowledge and truth of how to nourish your body with Protein Pacing and The PRISE Life fitness routines. You deserve this information to jet-set you to a new level of health and optimal performance that you will feel, see and start doing in every aspect of your life. This means you may notice the time you spend with your family and friends will be more enjoyable and active, and your time with coworkers will be more engaging and fulfilling, resulting in greater productivity. Most of all, your relationship with yourself and with others will be more meaningful and satisfying and your overall energy and outlook on life will be greatly enhanced. From T.F. Hodge, "The sky is not my limit… I am".

My commitment to you: I will always be here to support you on your PRISE Life journey, and this includes helping you build your own tribe of PRISE Life followers so we can bring this message to the world. Jump on board and let's change the world together . . . one PRISE Life at a time!

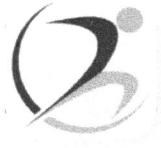

The Research
BEHIND REAL RESULTS

CHAPTER 8

SLOW, WHOLE AND DIRTY

A human body is a conversation going on, both within the cells and between the cells, and they're telling each other to grow and to die; when you're sick, something's gone wrong with that conversation.
— W. Daniel Hillis

Nourishing the body and nourishing the soul are the constants we as human beings need to work on throughout our lifetimes. It is a daily process, and we need to remain vigilant because if we let too much time go by without doing both, our quality of life suffers. This is why I am passionate about nurturance, with all its different facets, and committed to making sure the truth behind the science is revealed to you.

By presenting the facts from my research, I want to help you learn to listen to your body, to "mind" your body, and encourage you to follow The PRISE Life Protocol to help you become healthier and stronger and to achieve optimal health. As a result, you will probably exceed the performance level you initially dreamed of. This chapter will help you to be armed with some basic working knowledge, from an actual scientist who has spent years researching in a lab, of how nutrition works and, most importantly, what it means to actually nourish ourselves. *Hint: It is not with the plastic-covered chemical concoctions, microwaved and fast foods, or other processed things that we consume while washing them down with diet soft drinks and other "energy drinks."*

THE EPIDEMIC OF OBESITY

Many people today are not happy with their weight and are classified as obese—an alarming epidemic growing internationally—not only because of what they consume, or because of their lack of exercise, but also because of the lack of actual nutrients in what they are eating. We are filling our "hunger" with nutritionless products, and our bodies just can't figure out how to work properly, forget efficiently. It has become such an epidemic that the term malobesity has been coined. It refers to the individual who is malnourished due to heavy empty calories but has excess body fat (obesity). This epidemic didn't even exist twenty years ago.

When I look at the population today, it tugs at my heartstrings because there is no need for this much illness in the world. Stress is a major health risk for people of all ages, as demonstrated by increasing levels of the stress hormone cortisol. Cortisol is released when our internal hormonal system is triggered, such as during fight or flight situations. Unfortunately, the world we live in is delivering more and more fight or flight episodes throughout our day, and this is not healthy. In fact, higher levels of cortisol in our blood is associated with poor blood sugar control, and it is increasing our risk for a host of metabolic and heart-related illnesses By consuming large amounts of highly processed, high-calorie, prepackaged foods, we fail to get the nutrients, vitamins, and minerals we need for optimal body function. We are silently killing ourselves. This toxic food environment leads to excess weight gain, stress, and increased risk for all sorts of diseases. I'm here to say we are most definitely missing the key ingredient to a nutrition, fitness and emotional well-being protocol, and to point out where and why the errors are happening so you can give your beautiful body a chance to heal and even thrive again. There is no life when your days are wracked with pain and illness, or when you have difficulty breathing or moving. When you've tried every diet and exercise program out there and still can't seem to get any better, or even lose a few pounds, no wonder you feel defeated. I feel defeated for you.

And you are not solely to blame.

I don't want you to suffer another day. My heart can't take it! I want you to understand what metabolism and the body are all about so you can make permanent changes and enjoy all the fantastic things a healthy body has to offer.

Understand that a lack of nourishment, along with a lack of quality exercise, are why so many people are overweight and sick. We live in what we think is an educated world, and we have quick access to information that can easily be disseminated, but with misinformation so readily available, we are quickly getting sicker. And that is scary.

THE CRISIS OF HEALTH CARE

America is experiencing a strange paradox of sorts when it comes to health care. We are a nation that spends billions on pharmaceuticals to help solve many ills, yet we have pressing issues with alcohol and drug abuse, from heroin, to marijuana, to oxycodone. We are falling rapidly into the lower percentile of nations—nineteenth according to the World Health Organization—when it comes to good health and medical care. The U.S. spends 18% of its gross domestic product (GDP) on health-care, a higher proportion than any other country, but ranks 37th out of 191 countries according to its performance, which is beyond sad. Life expectancy is actually decreasing. Somehow, we are making the same poor health decisions every day despite spending an enormous amount of money on health care.

How could that be, you may ask, because you follow the government-recommended heart-healthy diet. You might think, Who am I supposed to believe? Do I trust the low-fat, heart-healthy diets; the low-carb, high-protein, and fat diets that encourage eating red meat, butter, bacon, and full cream; the high-fiber, high-carb diets; or the no-meat, vegetable-only diet? Or do you try the gluten-free, Paleo, ketogenic, fat-adapted, low-carb, low-fat, USDA My Plate, MIND, Mayo, plant-based, veganism, Atkins, DASH, Mediterranean, Weight Watchers, Plant Paradox, Jenny Craig, Metabolic Code, Volumetrics, Ornish, Flat Belly, Nutrisystem, Slimfast, South Beach, Zone, Acid-Alkaline, Fast, Raw/Macrobiotic, Dukan, or Whole30 diets, and on and on. You get it. There are so many to choose from, it's no wonder most people are utterly confused.

That's why I am here. In Chapter 3, I shared the most effective way to eat for optimal health and performance, with Protein Pacing. In this chapter, I'll share with you what I call the "Slow and Dirty Rules for Optimal Health." This will help you understand more completely what healthy eating really looks like.

THE FAST FOOD PARADOX

Recently, people have been talking about "slow" versus "fast" food, and my brother-in-law reminded me that not everyone is familiar with this concept. I've been a proponent of the "slow food" philosophy for years, but more people are familiar with the term "ast food. Essentially, fast food is exactly what the name implies—food that's been (mass) produced faster than its natural life cycle through the use of artificial stimulants such as fertilizers, over/forced-feeding methods, pesticides, hormones, growth factors, and genetically modified organisms.

Fast food includes food that comes in a "clean" wrapped package and is highly processed. This type of fast food often appears sterile, refined, and shiny and is referred to as "clean" food. Some health professionals confuse "eating clean" with eating healthy. However, "clean" applies much better to the fast-food production process and should be minimized. Fast food is the main staple in fast-food restaurants and convenience stores, but it's also abundant in traditional grocery stores. Fast food may also come in the form of conventional produce (fruits, vegetables, grains), animal products (milk, eggs, meat, etc.) and just about every prepackaged, processed food. Whatever the shape, size, and type of fast food, it's usually been mass-produced in tightly confined living quarters, such as a cage or feedlot, or in high-yield single-crop farms. Ironically, the shortened and stimulated production life cycle of fast food results in a strangely prolonged shelf life, once the food is harvested and brought to market. In other words, fast food is produced quickly but lives long. (Think of the Twinkie with the urban legend twenty-plus-year shelf life!)

Herein lies the hidden danger of fast food. The longer-than-normal shelf life wreaks havoc on the human body, because the harmful chemicals used to protect and stimulate the growth of the vegetable, fruit, grain, or animal gets passed on to the cells in our body. Many experts believe these synthetic chemicals contribute to the current plague of modern-day diseases, such as cardiovascular and metabolic disease, certain cancers, as well as inflammatory and neurodegenerative disorders. I call it the "fast-food paradox"—a shortened life cycle and prolonged shelf life (afterlife). Disturbingly, a recent analysis by the World Wide Fund concluded that the average person ingests the equivalent of a credit card amount of plastic per week . . . (that's a lot of phthalates . . . yuck!) In reality, toxins are everywhere, and I will discuss this topic in much greater detail later in the book. In the meantime, pay attention to the quality of the food you eat now!

EAT SLOW

We've all been told at some point that eating slow is good for our digestion and our health. However, slow food is the opposite of fast food. It includes foods that have been grown and raised without the use of harmful toxins and artificial growth factors and protectants, and thus require a longer life cycle to grow and mature. Once these foods have undergone their natural course of growth, their shelf life is usually very short.

Examples of slow food include local and/or organic produce, free-range, grass-fed beef, dairy, eggs, and poultry, as well as most wild seafood. You're probably thinking, if it's local, it must be "fast." Actually, local produce (vegetables and fruits) and animal-based products mature according to the timeline that nature intended. Therefore, it comes to the market, and eventually your dinner table, long after conventional food sources arrive.

Slow food is characterized by an extended, natural life cycle and a brief shelf life (afterlife), so you need to restock more often. This is a good thing. As such, there is limited, if any, exposure to harmful toxic residues entering our cells. Slow food is rich in nutrients and other healthy chemicals called antioxidants and polyphenolic compounds, all of which protect our bodies from disease.

EAT DIRTY

Local farmers' markets, community-supported agriculture (CSA), home gardens/farms, and clean oceans and freshwater streams/lakes are ideal sources for much of your staple food items. These are also where you will find the healthiest sources of "dirty" whole foods. "Dirty" foods are those foods that come directly from the earth and sea—think vegetables, grains, beans, fruits, seeds/nuts, and animal foods (fish, meat, eggs, dairy). Because these foods are grown in the earth, they sometimes even come with a little dirt still on them! This is a good thing! This is a healthy thing!

At any moment during the day, you have a choice between nutrient-dense slow and dirty food, including nutrient-dense engineered food, or fast food. I want you to do everything in your power to choose nutrient-dense slow and dirty food and eat it often.

WHOLE FOOD VS. ENGINEERED FOOD

Growing your own food from the earth's soil is ultimately the greatest source of nourishment to keep our bodies healthy and functioning at the highest level. Mother Earth is, undoubtedly, still the prime nourisher, and if we focus on the quality of unadulterated soil and nutrients found within, as originally created, we as a species will thrive again. The problem is that the soils are so depleted and we are eating so much genetically modified and manufactured foods that often contain high levels of toxins, that we have to replace the nutrients that have been taken away from us. We have to focus on high-quality (whole) foods to become a healthier world.

The pressing question, and one you are probably wondering about is, "What about these new packaged nutritional diets? Are they even good for me?" To keep you motivated, and onboard, I want to comment. I believe we can obtain optimal nourishment from high-quality whole foods as well as powders, bars, and meal replacements that contain naturally sourced high-quality raw ingredients. I refer to this as "nutrient-dense engineered" food as opposed to "nutrient-deficient engineered" food (that is loaded with artificial sweeteners or refined sugar, sodium and lacking in fiber and nutrients).

Some would say all meat, vegetables, fruits, dairy, etc. are whole foods, so they must be good for us; however, the manner in which they are grown (heavy pesticides, insecticides, etc.), cultivated (genetically modified organism [GMO], etc.), and cared for (caged, grain-fed, etc.) make a huge difference and sometimes are less healthy than high-quality "packaged goods," meal replacements, and supplements or "nutrient-dense engineered" foods. I know the quality of a certain few nutritional-supplement companies that source the best ingredients in their bars, powders, meal replacements, vitamins/minerals, etc., that are of higher quality than many "whole foods." After years of research and personal interest, I have found the ones that truly can step up your health with the proper and needed combinations of complementary vitamins, minerals, and phytonutrients (plant nutrients). They are not packed with sugar, and they don't just throw in a smidgen of an ingredient to be able to make fancy claims. Find out which bars, powders, meal replacements, and supplements I recommend in The PRISE Life app, The PRISE Life Facebook page, and in The PRISE Life Cookbook.

Now that I've thrown at you trying to eat slow and dirty food, whole foods, and the fact that I am not against nutritional supplementation and meal replacements, and in case I've overwhelmed you, here is the great news: To achieve optimal health, you need your cells to be nurtured, and any changes you make on a daily basis with this philosophy are going to pay off. One less diet soda, one less fast food, one less high-calorie, sodium-rich, prepackaged meal, one well-documented and researched healthier supplementation product, one less sugar- and caffeine-packed energy drink, and you are on your way to creating healthier habits that will pay off in the near future.

A wonderful side effect of this new type of eating is that soon you are going to find the taste of fake food and smell of fake scents "off," and you will start craving more flavorful, earth-based, healthful food and natural essences. How fun that finally "dirty" is a good word. These small steps alone are going to help your metabolism and body's healing in ways you would never believe.

GO AHEAD AND CHEAT

Another finding of my research, and one I think you will like, is that you can cheat! I'm one of the first scientists to include a "cheat day" in my research studies, with phenomenal results! I did this because I will be the first person to say, perfection is impossible, and allowing ourselves the occasional treat when it comes to food is one way to keep us on track.

In my PRISE Life Cookbook, I detail my 85%–15% Rule. This simply means try to eat healthy and dirty foods 85% of the time, and the other 15% of the time indulge in your favorite comfort foods. To make this even easier to follow using my Protein Pacing plan, simply include one "cheat meal" a day, or set aside one day each week to indulge. Either way, this adheres to my 85%–15% Rule. But remember, stay within the same number of total calories for each "cheat meal or day" that you would normally follow.

EATING TO CLEANSE OUR BODIES OF TOXINS

Now that you know more about the health benefits of slow food and eating dirty, I want you to think of other products you may be using that expose your body to toxins. It could be the crazy "clean" concoctions in shampoo or skin cream. It could be "fresh and clean" scented air fresheners, cleaning products, toothpaste, you name it. Many of our personal care and household products are filled with chemicals that may harm, not heal, your body. They are just as dangerous to your cells as the foods we ingest.

The wonderful news is that my research shows that following the Protein Pacing eating plan, along with intermittent fasting (described in the next chapter), increases the rate at which you expel toxins. I am pretty much the first to discuss the relationship between weight loss, toxins, and oxidative stress through scientific measures. It is exciting to realize that we now have scientific evidence that the quality of your diet does matter! Through diet, we can favorably support the detoxification process, oxidative stress levels, and blood vessel health, all while enhancing weight loss.

This major study of mine, in particular, was cited by *Science Daily* on January 11, 2017, which stated, "*Research by exercise scientists has found that a balanced, protein-pacing, low-calorie diet that includes intermittent fasting not only achieves long-term weight loss but also helps release toxins in the form of polychlorinated biphenyls (PCBs) from the body fat stores, in addition to enhancing heart health and reducing oxidative stress.*" In case you don't know what and how detrimental they are, PCBs are a group of organic compounds used in the manufacture of plastics, as lubricants, and dielectric fluids in transformers, in protective coating for wood, metal, and concrete, and in adhesives, wire coating, and so forth. They are highly toxic to aquatic life and persist in the environment for long periods of time. They can accumulate in food chains and may produce harmful side effects at high concentrations. The extent to which our world has become contaminated by these is mind-boggling. Other common contaminants in our food supply include phthalates, which are highly toxic and disease promoting.

We know we need to reduce exposure to these toxins, but how proactive are we about this? Have we become complacent because we are too tired to care? Or have we just become frozen, unable to move because we have no clue as to the direction that is best for our bodies, especially with all the latest and greatest diets coming out? Well, I am here to share some amazing news and to unparalyze you!

With the smallest of efforts by humans to improve their own miraculous creation, by eating a certain way, what we found was that the body actually compensated, took over, and worked on its own by increasing disease-fighting antioxidants and decreasing cellular-damaging oxidative stress.

This is astounding. In response to this flood of PCBs that were being released from their storage sites, the fat cells (called adipocytes), especially the visceral abdominal fat cells, the body was coming to its own defense, likely scavenging and squelching the toxins. It is because of this that we had a healthy weight-loss intervention for all the participants in the research study. This is an important public health message, and it is being missed in a lot of the fad diets used out there. It is yet another reason why my PRISE Protocol that includes Protein Pacing and intermittent nutritional fasting will last long after others have been forgotten—but you will want to follow it precisely. No reinventing the wheel needed. It is designed to help your body release toxins from your stored body fat, especially the visceral abdominal fat, which in turn will help you lose weight and feel great.

CONCLUSION

Always remember that at the core, say yes to slow, whole and dirty foods, and yes to nutrient-dense engineered food, and no to clean, refined, prepackaged, "nutrient-deficient" chemical foods. Your body will help you release toxins quicker than you might have ever believed. Let's really commit to nourishing our bodies and finally let the cells have a healthy communication chain. With clear, natural, and healing channels, a dramatic change and increased vitality are bound to bless you. I promise you, by implementing these small steps, even the weakest bodies can start to unclog, detox, and get healthy. With the slow, whole and dirty food knowledge ingrained in your subconscious, nudging you to do what is right, we will now move on to fasting, juicing and proteins.

CHAPTER 9

THE TRUTH ABOUT FASTING, JUICING AND PROTEINS

The best of all medicines are resting and fasting.
— *Benjamin Franklin*

One very popular lifestyle strategy that has gained enormous attention is intermittent fasting, sometimes referred to as intermittent nutritional fasting or nutritionally supported cleanse. Specifically, intermittent fasting is often associated with helping the body restore, replenish, rejuvenate, and heal, and recently has even shown signs of slowing down aging in humans. This is referred to as autophagy, or the removal of damaged cellular structures. The reason is our bodies naturally go through cycles of breaking down and building up as well as periodic "house cleaning." The ideal scenario/environment for the body to perform its house cleaning is similar to the process we use in our own homes. The best time to house clean is when there is not a lot of clutter, basically an empty house. Inside our bodies, intermittent fasting is associated with the best environment to clean house and restore optimal function.

Intermittent fasting can be accomplished in several different ways:

- **16/8 Method:** Consists of fasting for sixteen hours (no food or caloric drinks, only water) and then eating two or more meals within an eight-hour window. Also called time-restricted feeding or eating (TRF).

- **5:2 Method:** Involves five days of normal eating and two days of fasting that limits calorie intake to 300–600 calories. The two-day fasts can be any two days during the week.

- **24-Hour Fast Method:** This is the typical fast most people are familiar with, which involves refraining from eating and drinking (water only) up to 500 calories for a twenty-four-hour period one to two days per week.

- **Alternate Day Fasting Method:** As the name implies, this requires fasting every other day either with no food (water only) or eating up to 500 calories during the fast days.

There are other modifications of these four main types of fasting, such as the fasting-mimicking diet, that are the most well-known and followed. While they each provide a slightly different form of intermittent fasting, the 5:2 and 24-Hour Fast methods provide the best environment to achieve the best results, if done properly.

If your goal is weight loss, incorporate the 5:2 or 24-Hour Fast methods on a weekly basis for up to three months. Once you've achieved your weight loss goal, aim to fast only one to two days per month. If you're not interested in weight loss, reap the benefits of either of these methods by fasting one to two days per month. This is the exact intermittent fasting routine I've used in my own research with fantastic results!

GUIDELINES FOR SUCCESSFUL FASTING

The quality of the 300–600 calories you consume on these intermittent fasting days will make or break the benefit it provides your body. In other words, paying close attention to ingesting high-quality, nutrient-dense, phytochemical (antioxidant/adaptogen-rich) foods is the key to getting the best results. I have the published research to support this!

Some of the best sources of antioxidants (substances that prevent damaging oxidative stress reactions in the body) and adaptogens (plant substances that help our bodies adapt to stress) I've used in my research to support intermittent nutritional fasting, include: blueberries, raspberries, bilberries, turmeric, rhodiola, ashwagandha, bacopa, schizandra, eleuthero, and pau d'arco.

Here is a simple and very effective 1-2 day/week intermittent nutritional fast (or cleanse) I've used with clients, athletes, and study participants:

Before breakfast:	multivitamin with adaptogen beverage (25 calories)
Breakfast:	antioxidant beverage with protein snack (70 calories)
Mid-morning snack:	small handful of nuts/seeds and dried fruit (50 calories for women, 100 calories for men)
Lunch:	antioxidant beverage with protein snack (70 calories)
Mid-afternoon snack:	antioxidant beverage with protein snack (70 calories for women, 120 calories for men)
Dinner:	antioxidant beverage with protein snack and multivitamin (70 calories)

This intermittent fast cleanse provides about 350 calories for women and 450 calories for men per day.

Some people like to use the term cleansing to identify this intermittent fasting period of very-low-calorie intake that allows the body to fully and properly remove harmful or unwanted substances (toxins) that have accumulated. I know it's a funny analogy, but as I said, the same way it is easiest and most effective to clean an empty house, it's also most effective to clean out and restore our bodies to optimal health when there is less food and less junk in it.

This Protein Pacing program does not ask people to deprive themselves for long periods of time, and it does not ask a diabetic with a blood sugar-issue not to eat. This program is about nourishing the body to a point that when the healthy foods, and possible supplements, are added, they are not just flushed out of the body with all the other goop that has built up in the bowels or even in the organs and tissues.

THE BENEFITS AND METHODS OF JUICING

When we think of cleaning out our bodies, people also often mix the words juicing with cleansing, so I want to address this. As a young boy, I remember using a spinning juicer with freshly squeezed oranges and grapefruits during the cold winter months—the juice was delicious and always seemed to keep our house of nine people living in close quarters a bit healthier than our friends and neighbors! These days, juicing is all the rage in nutrition and health. But what is juicing, and is it really better for us than the real deal of fresh fruits and vegetables? Essentially, juicing is the process of extracting only the juice-containing portion of any fruit or vegetable, leaving behind the outer (skin) layer, seeds, and most of the pulp and natural fiber. This results in a liquid-rich cornucopia of health-promoting vitamins, minerals, and other potent bioactive compounds, also known as PHYTO (plant-based) chemicals. The most well-known of these phytochemicals are antioxidants, which are often associated with powerful health benefits such as increased immunity and disease protection, as well as enhanced energy.

There are two main juice-extraction methods: heat-generated and cold-pressed. The heat-generating juicers use a super-fast spinning blade (called centrifugal extractors) against a mesh filter that separates the pulp from the juice. The limitation of these juicers is that they produce a lot of heat while spinning, which likely destroys the natural enzymes within the fruit and vegetables as well as oxidizes some of the health-promoting nutrients.

The cold-pressed method of juicing, on the other hand, is considered much gentler because it simply crushes and then presses the fruit and vegetables, retaining nearly all the enzymes and other health-boosting phytochemicals (antioxidants). As a result, the takeaway message from many juicing pundits is that cold-pressed is a healthier choice, and I agree.

Both heat-generated and cold-pressed juices are susceptible to spoilage due to microorganism growth. This limits their shelf life to two to five days, at most. So drink up quickly! Heat pasteurization methods are often used to neutralize the harmful microorganisms that lead to spoilage, which extends the juice life up to forty-five days. However, there is a downside to pasteurization. Similar to heat-generated juice extraction, heat-pasteurization destroys many of the health-promoting properties of the fruit or vegetable juice.

Recently, a new processing technique has been introduced to the juicing market that neutralizes harmful micro-organisms and similarly extends juice life up to forty-five days, but without the negative consequences of typical heat-generated pasteurization. This process is referred to as high-pressure processing, or HPP. According to recent food science research, HPP retains many of the original nutrients, flavor, and texture of fruits and vegetables (HPP versus thermal pasteurization). This is reason enough to always choose fresh juices that have been prepared using both cold-pressed and HPP techniques instead of standard heat processing and pasteurization methods.

Most food science experts agree that eating the whole fruit or vegetable, especially a local and/or organic version, should be your top priority for optimal health. But let's face it, our hectic on-the-go lifestyles place convenience at a premium. As such, the quick, convenient, and long shelf life of cold-pressed, HPP juices provide a nourishing alternative to the real deal. But if you want to enjoy the highest level of nourishment on the go, opt for a whole fruit and vegetable-blended smoothie with some added protein. This will provide all of the vitamins, minerals, antioxidants, fiber, and other nutrients contained within the whole fruit and vegetable and will save you money too. Although the whole fruit and vegetable protein smoothie may provide a bit more calories, the fiber and roughage will benefit you more in the end. In those weak or on-the-run moments, choose the whole fruit and nothing but the fruit as often as you can.

PROTEIN POWDERS

With our house cleaned and juicing addressed, I want to discuss the most important part of my program: PROTEIN. There are more healthy types of protein out there than you may have been led to believe and some of them are newer.

Normally when we think of protein we think only of animal products, but you will learn that plant sources, including vegetables, grains, nuts, and legumes have protein too. Even some of the newer created sources, like protein powders, provide excellent sources of protein. Since the invention of these powders and the actual understanding that plants have protein, I recommend them, and even prefer them in some circumstances. However, and this is a big beware, quality is everything. If the powders come from good sources of animal foods like whey or collagen, or from plant sources like pea, brown rice, fava, mung, pumpkin seed, tapioca, legumes, or hemp (and some forms of soy) protein, they can help support an excellent diet. But if they are full of simple and/or fake sugars, have mismatched nutrients thrown in, are too small to have any health benefit, or are topped with artificial flavorings and preservatives, run for your life! These types are no better than gulping down a fast-food burger and mistakenly thinking that you are nourishing yourself! Chances are, you will also be hungry about fifteen minutes after you just finished that meal.

I always ask myself, "Protein powder, but at what cost?"

DAIRY PROTEINS

The first and perhaps most popular protein powder source these days is called whey protein.

But what is whey? Remember Mother Goose? "Little Miss Muffet, sat on a tuffet, Eating her curds and whey." Do you know what this is? It is the lumps and liquid of nothing other than cottage cheese! Yup! And guess what the clumping parts are? Protein curds. And the liquid part? Whey! Now don't say Mother Goose wasn't trying to teach us something! But all joking aside, whey proteins are the byproduct—the waste product—that occurs in the production of cheese, which, of course, comes from milk. A great resource is *The Dairy Processing Handbook,* which states that "Milk is made of two proteins: casein and whey. Whey protein can be separated from the casein in milk or formed as a byproduct of cheese making." It is important to note that, "Whey protein is considered a complete protein, as it contains all nine essential amino acids (and 11 non-essential amino acids). It is low in lactose content." We will have more on this in the next chapter on macronutrients, but for now let's focus on lactose, the sugar component of dairy.

A lot of people have issues with dairy, or rather the lactose in dairy, and therefore as these powders have evolved, so has the level of lactose in them. That's why you might have heard terms like concentrate vs. isolate vs. hydrolysate. All this has been created because now you can remove lactose from whey through a process called filtration. This process makes even the lactose intolerant able to use some whey protein.

Filtration is a widespread method used in the creation of whey protein powders, and when handled correctly can result in all, but 15% of the lactose being successfully extracted from the whey. The ion-exchange process is less affordable and may result in a final product that has all but 5% of the lactose removed. If you really want to get into the nitty-gritty of the process, I recommend *The Dairy Processing Handbook*, and the chapter on "Whey Processing." But I'm going to share the major points in lay people's terms, so let's start with the concentrate.

TYPES OF WHEY PROTEIN

Whey protein concentrate is slightly less filtered, and therefore less processed than whey protein isolate or hydrolysate. It is usually about 80% protein (watch the brand because some are as low as 35% and use unhealthy fillers). Remember, a higher percentage of protein is better because it is higher protein by weight. But beware, if you are lactose intolerant, this may still give you problems because there is inherently a larger concentration of lactose in a concentrate. The upside is you are going to have the best immune-boosting support from this least-processed form, and it digests more slowly so it keeps you satiated longer and contains health-boosting micro/macroglobulin proteins and peptides.

If the concentrate is treated more, it becomes the second stage and 90% pure protein by weight, often even 95%. Isolate protein supplements undergo several purification processes that filter out virtually all of the fat and carbohydrates, and because of this are about 95% pure protein by weight. The benefits of whey protein isolate are that it is easily digestible, contains very low amounts of lactose, and also increases protein synthesis, allowing for a large spike in amino acid levels. The healthy micro/macroglobulin proteins and peptides in concentrate are not present in isolate, and therefore whey protein concentrate is actually considered healthier by many experts than isolate. Almost all the lactose is removed, so it is good for lactose intolerance, but because it is broken into smaller peptides, you may lose some immune-boosting benefits.

Hydrolyzed protein (hydrolysate) was created to remove the allergenic issues for people and also provide the highest amount of protein per volume. It is also the fastest absorbing type of whey protein because it is already so broken down. Many hard-core bodybuilding and fitness models opt for this, but it's not my top choice in terms of overall health benefits because the process destroys most of the immune benefits.

You may have heard of undenatured and denatured whey protein. Essentially, undenatured means the naturally occurring proteins and bioactive compounds have not been altered with chemicals and high-temperature heating during processing. Whereas, denatured whey protein has been chemically altered, and, therefore the health-promoting compounds have been destroyed in an attempt to produce a more highly concentrated form of whey protein. Based on the available scientific evidence, I recommend undenatured whey protein concentrate. This type of whey protein is in its most natural form and yields many of the health benefits it was intended to provide from nature. Choosing an undenatured whey protein that is natural-eco-sourced from grass-fed or pasture-raised cows may add further benefit by providing a higher concentration and amount of heart and health-boosting omega-3 fatty acids.

In the laboratory, we actually spend time looking and talking about something called the biological value (BV) of protein sources. BV measures how efficiently a protein source is digested, and after that used in protein synthesis. If all the protein you digest from a certain source is made available to the body to make different proteins, it's incredibly effective and receives a high BV score. The less protein from a certain source that may be made available for protein synthesis receives a lower score. It's fascinating to note that whey protein isolate has a BV score of about 160—the highest BV score of any protein source known to man to date.

THE CASE FOR CASEIN PROTEIN

Raw cow's milk is 5%–10% protein, out of which 80% is casein and 20% whey. Like whey, casein protein has a high BV value (BV of 90) that suggests it contains all the essential amino acids required for protein synthesis in your body. Casein is a slow-digesting protein, meaning it takes longer to enter the bloodstream and cells and initiate protein synthesis compared to whey protein, which is very fast acting. The speed of the gastric emptying slows down, meaning acids in casein enter the blood more slowly. Just one scoop of casein (also called micellar) protein contains a massive 24g of protein. Casein allows for the repair and healing of muscle fibers to reduce muscle soreness and increase protein synthesis. Through helping shorten healing time, casein protein can help you increase power and strength and allow you to train harder. By consuming casein, you may get a great source of protein without excess calories, including carbohydrates. Studies show that casein protein may promote weight reduction and decrease excess fat.

You may want to consider taking casein protein before bed. This type of protein is often recommended as the best nighttime meal. Scientific research shows casein protein may take up to seven hours to digest, which is just about as long as the common person sleeps every night. Casein extends the release of amino acids into the bloodstream, improving protein (nitrogen) retention and thus the ability to build muscle. Any period spent sleeping is a period when your body is not getting any new nutrients. If you run out of amino acids in your bloodstream, your body can start breaking down muscle proteins to fuel itself. Taking casein before going to bed is an effective strategy to avoid protein breakdown and amino acid oxidation.

So which is best for muscle development or lean body composition, whey or casein? It really depends on your overall goal. If optimal health and peak performance are your top priority, I recommend undenatured whey protein concentrate. If you are solely focused on muscle development, then include both casein and whey protein. Because there is controversy regarding the health effects of casein protein, always have some source of undenatured whey concentrate in your diet. Casein in milk consists of both A1 and A2 beta-casein proteins. Research shows that milk containing A1 beta-casein is associated with intolerances and gastro-intestinal discomfort such as bloating, gas, diarrhea and inflammation compared to milk that contains only A2 beta-casein. Therefore, A1 beta-casein containing milk should be avoided and only A2 beta-casein milk should be consumed. In my opinion, whey is the healthier choice between the two and should be the primary form of your protein intake combined with healthy plant-based sources.

DR. PAUL'S FAVORITE PLANT-BASED PROTEIN

I'm a huge plant-based protein supporter because of the many proven health and performance benefits of eating a plant-based diet. Having said this, I also want to clearly point out that our bodies respond more favorably to animal-based protein when it comes to lean muscle mass and fat burning. That's just science, and is why most of the research supports animal-based protein to maximize body composition. However, plant-based protein provides awesome health benefits such as antioxidants, fiber, vitamins, minerals, and delicious goodness that make us feel completely nourished.

Of all the plant-based proteins, a combination of pea, almond, pecan, tiger nuts, fava, mung, sesame seed, pumpkin seed, flaxseed, pine nut, pistachio, hemp, and brown rice protein are some of the highest quality (with other plant-based proteins like fermented soy showing some health and body composition benefits). Eating these in powder form is a healthy and effective way to meet your Protein Pacing goals, and I enjoy these myself. Of course, whole food plant-based proteins are excellent sources, and should be consumed daily. However, you'll do best to avoid soy protein powders because of the processing and higher levels of plant estrogens (phytoestrogens). Instead, choose other plant-based powders as well as certain animal proteins such as whey and collagen bone broth protein for their proven health benefits. If you consume soy protein, stay with naturally occurring whole plant sources, such as fermented soy (tofu), edamame, tempeh, miso, and natto.

Unfortunately, a great deal of controversy surrounds the intake of healthy complex carbohydrates such as grains (rice, barley, quinoa, oats, spelt, rye, kashi, corn) vegetables/fruits (potatoes, peppers, pumpkin, squash, wheatgrass, citrus fruits, melons, etc.) and legumes (lentils, chickpeas, black beans, kidney beans, etc.) because they contain the anti-nutrient 'lectin' protein. In fact, many popular diet "fad" books wrongly accuse lectin as the primary reason for obesity, inflammation and poor digestive health when in fact, there is very little human scientific evidence for lectins causing these conditions. This is because, most lectins found in raw plants, such as legumes, squashes, pumpkins, and most grains are rarely eaten uncooked. Cooking and/or soaking the plants deactivates most of the lectin. In support of this, cultures that regularly consume high intakes of these grains, plants and legumes are some of the healthiest populations in the world.

PROTEIN POWDER CONCLUSION

The bottom line is that undenatured whey concentrate is the best protein powder source. Remember that quality is everything. Whey is a complete protein with amino acids that can turn on protein synthesis and thereby help the muscles and bones/body thrive. Using the right amount at the right time can help you lose weight and gain lean muscle mass, and it's one of my top go-tos for Protein Pacing. It has vital nutrients, and it opens up so many protein options for you to consume that your meals will never get boring and you will stay full longer.

I hope this discussion of intermittent fasting, juicing, "house cleaning," biological value of protein, and whey vs. plant proteins such as soy and legumes help you feel more confident about the choices you make every day. In the end, I don't want the truth annihilated or only partial truths told. I am hopeful that my views, with scientific proof to back them up, will help you have the energy to continue to think critically and make the right and informed choices for you and your loved ones. Now let's take a look at how our bodies metabolize the food we eat.

CHAPTER 10

HUMAN
METABOLISM 101

While weight loss is important, what's more important is the
quality of food you put in your body—food is information
that quickly changes your metabolism and genes.
— Mark Hyman, MD

It is amazing to me that Human Metabolism 101 is not taught as early as middle school. How our body functions should be a necessary course in how to live, eat, and survive. This is one of the reasons I've made it a point to visit elementary, middle, and high schools throughout my thirty-year career and help educate young people on metabolism and the benefits of healthy eating and proper fitness. I even made the news for going to Washington, DC, and Capitol Hill to speak directly to legislators about the importance of maintaining the funding from the National Institute of Health for Heart Disease Research and Stroke Prevention and then for the school lunch program. I want to make sure we have adequate funding and programs in place so that our children are fed healthy food while at school. It was an exciting and eye-opening trip!

ACCURATE INFORMATION MATTERS

There are many fascinating hidden facts about the human body, which is why I have invested all these years researching and teaching. Did you know that even when your body is at rest, it requires energy for the functioning of organs, breathing, circulating the blood, contracting the heart, adjusting bodily hormone levels, and growing and repairing cells? The rate of energy consumed by the body at rest is known as the basal metabolic rate, or BMR.

Much of my early research as a nutrition and exercise scientist studied BMR, or the more current term, resting metabolic rate (RMR), and I soon became known as the "Metabolism Doctor." To this day, I remain humbled and honored to have contributed much of our current understanding of metabolism based on my scientific research findings in women and men of varying ages, health status, and fitness levels.

Many health books and quick-fix diet books talk about metabolism, healthy eating, and proper fitness. My goal is to not only refresh your memory, but to help you debunk some of the latest and craziest theories or misinformation out there. My research was touted for its effectiveness in Fox News Lifestyle, with an article titled, "How to get into the best shape of your life, according to science!" Another exciting moment in my career! I've studied and researched what I share. There is no guessing in my protocols and advice. Let's dive in!

ASSIMILATING NUTRIENTS, RELEASING TOXINS

Metabolism is a complex biochemical process in which food is converted into energy so our bodies can function. Metabolism is much more than just gaining or losing weight, as some "experts" have led us to believe. Metabolism is the engine that keeps us going. It's simple to understand with a car that we can't put sugar in a gas engine because it kills it, permanently. Well, the food we put into our bodies, for our metabolism engine, determines how fast and how far we can run, and how long we can last. We are living beings that need actual nutrients from the food we eat to convert into energy, or we simply stop functioning and get sick or die.

Metabolism also performs a vital role in our bodies of cleaning our "house" and releasing toxins, as discussed in Chapter 9. This often-missed function of metabolism is the reason why some people who are following a calorie-restricted diet—maybe even pushing their bodies too strenuously with exercise— are still NOT losing weight. We are faced daily with poisons, contaminants, toxins, pesticides, drugs, and even alcohol, and these damaging substances need to be removed from the body so that the nutrients in our food can be properly absorbed and converted into energy. It is important to not only nourish our body with proper foods, but to also "clean house" and restore the body by releasing these toxins we encounter every day. This is essential for our cells to have a shot at functioning optimally.

THE ROLE OF HORMONES IN HEALTH AND WEIGHT LOSS

A third function of metabolism is the important role of using specific proteins to properly control the chemical reactions of the metabolic process. Hormones produced by the organs (endocrine system) control the rate at which we can metabolize food. One of these hormones, thyroxine, produced and released by the thyroid, plays a key role in determining how quickly or slowly the chemical reactions of the metabolic processes occur within the body. When the body does not produce the correct amount of this hormone, the process of losing weight or gaining health gets a little more complicated, even with the proper healthy foods.

This is where the holistic and integrative approach of The PRISE Life Protocol, with Protein Pacing and the RISE fitness program, has the potential to unlock the magic within each of us, even those struggling with menopause.

THE EFFECTS OF STRESS AND CORTISOL

Cortisol is another hormone plaguing our bodies and our health. It is released from the adrenal glands in response to stress (think fight-or-flight response), which also causes sugar (glucose) to be released from the liver. Unfortunately, the more often we are exposed to stress and higher cortisol levels, the more our cells are exposed to higher blood sugar levels and become less sensitive to the hormone insulin. Insulin's primary role is to help shuttle glucose into our cells (muscle and fat), so when it's not doing its job well, blood sugar levels continue to rise and much of the excess sugar finds its way to our belly fat for storage.

In addition, our endocrine system (hormones) is being damaged by the harmful toxins around us such as polychlorinated biphenyls (PCBs), dioxins, phthalates, and dichloro diphenyl trichloroethane (DDT)—that first-of-its-kind synthetic insecticide introduced in the 1940s.

Despite this, I have good news. Once you start following The PRISE Life eating and cleansing protocol, your body will understand that it is healing. As the confused signals start to clear up and redirect the internal conversations (with the aid of the energy from the properly timed food and nutrients you are eating), your body will find the power to produce more energy and function more efficiently. As a result, it will offer you more strength, breathing power, and endurance—more health and life power to enjoy. Who doesn't dream of that?

THE IMPORTANCE OF BUILDUP AND BREAKDOWN

In expanding your knowledge of chemical reactions and the need for energy to flow, here is the next crucial concept of metabolism that I want you to understand and embrace: anabolism and catabolism. These are part of a natural cycle that exists perfectly in the human body. Think of the body's metabolism as a way to build up, break down, and build itself up again.

Anabolism is the constructive metabolic process that is the building and storing function of the metabolic process. It supports the growth of new cells, the maintenance of body tissues, and the storage of energy for future use, so it is the building-up phase. Catabolism is the destructive breaking-down metabolic process, which is the process that produces the energy required for all activities in the cells. During this phase of the biochemical process—through calories from carbohydrates, fats, and proteins, along with oxygen—it breaks down or releases the energy our bodies need to function.

Our bodies are complex but perfectly created, and with proper nutrition, we can help our bodies build up, break down, and build up again. With this concept alone, you will have learned more than most people know. How can we help the process? By carefully thinking about the food we put in our bodies. By carefully picking calories that nourish us, versus "empty" or harmful calories that have little or no nutrition, we will find that we feel more alert, more motivated, and happier.

EATING TO LOSE WEIGHT

When we are able to consistently nourish ourselves throughout the day with the right amount of nutrient-dense food, at set timing and intervals, we start to see how well we can truly function. It's amazing to think that fat or weight gain is often just a sign that your poor body has an energy imbalance, and it is trying to get you to pay attention. It is conversing with us, because as Mark Hyman says, "Food is information that quickly changes your metabolism and genes." The question is, are we listening?

As I've stressed, metabolism is far more complex than consuming fewer calories to lose more weight. Skipping meals, or regularly reducing caloric intake to under 500 calories a day, as some diets recommend, is not a wise choice. There is a lot of bad information out there, so beware.

When you cut calories that low, you are simply forcing your body into starvation mode to protect you, and your metabolic process will drastically slow to try to conserve energy and save your life. As a result, it will hold on to every calorie possible, giving you the opposite long-term result than what you are looking for—weight gain, especially fat gain, and with it, the potential to store and hold on to even more toxins! A body cannot survive without nourishment, and with too few calories consistently, especially without quality calories, your body will eventually shut down or starve to death.

A person with pounds and pounds of fat mass and a massive buildup in decomposing matter stuck in the intestines can also starve to death. So again, it goes back to making sure the body can find the time to break down, cleanse, restore, and rebuild itself. Remember the difference between intermittent fasting and starvation. The first is a "cleaning house" for better health and endurance; the second is depletion where you starve yourself to death, or at least become so malnourished that illness can take over. Your stomach will happily agree with me on this when it is growling away. I do NOT recommend long-term starvation diets!

BURN, BABY, BURN (CALORIES)

As an expert on the subject, I want to briefly explain the major components of our overall metabolism so you have a much clearer picture of how moment-by-moment lifestyle strategies may greatly benefit our health and fitness. As I said at the beginning of this chapter, even when your body is at rest it requires energy to function. This is known as the resting metabolic rate (RMR) and is the rate of energy consumed by the body at rest. The RMR is the energy that is just sufficient enough for the function of the body's tissues and vital organs. The largest component of our total daily metabolism, often referred to as our total daily energy expenditure (TDEE), is our RMR, because it accounts for roughly 60%–75% of the total number of calories we burn over the course of a day.

For example, if you burn 2,400 calories a day, your RMR would burn 1,440 calories (which is exactly 1 calorie burned per minute over a twenty-four-hour period—there are 1,440 minutes in a day) to as many as 1,800 calories. The remainder of the calories you burn during the day is the result of three primary metabolic processes:

Thermic Effect of Food   The calories we burn after we eat a meal, called the thermic effect of food (TEF), account for about 10% of our TDEE. In our example using 2,400 calories a day for our TDEE, the TEF would be 240 calories for digestion, absorption, transport, metabolism, storage, and excretion of food. *As I will discuss later, this can change drastically based on macronutrients (fats, carbohydrates, and proteins) and other foods/drinks we eat and when we eat them.*

Thermic Effect of Activity   The calories we burn due to physical activity and structured exercise, called the thermic effect of activity (TEA), is the most variable, as you can imagine. But for most of us, it ranges from 15%–30% of our TDEE, which would be 360–720 calories a day. This is equivalent to thirty to ninety minutes of walking, jogging, or running a day.

Non-Exercise Activity Thermogenesis   The calories we burn while we are NOT sleeping, eating, or exercising are what we refer to as non-exercise activity thermogenesis, or NEAT. This includes performing spontaneous movement, such as standing shivering, working on a computer or other device, and all forms of fidgeting or non-purposeful movements we routinely engage in that we may not even be aware of. This includes constantly shaking your legs while driving (which I do and which drives my wife bonkers!). NEAT also includes "air drumming" while watching TV or sitting in the back seat of the car (as our older son loves to do). This is all NEAT. Amazingly, NEAT can account for as little as 5%, or up to as much as 50% or more of TDEE! That's an enormous range of calories across a day, which can make huge impacts on health and physical performance. In our example, it's 120–1,200 calories!

Total Daily Energy Expenditure (Metabolism)

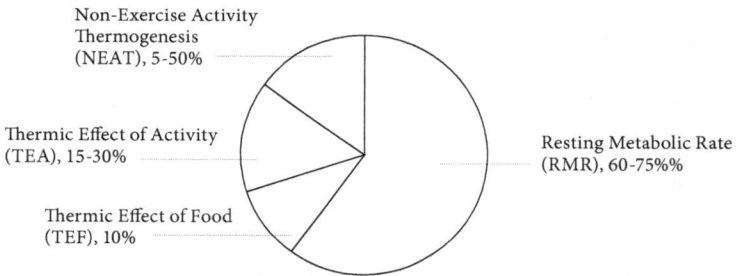

Non-Exercise Activity
Thermogenesis
(NEAT), 5-50%

Thermic Effect of Activity
(TEA), 15-30%

Thermic Effect of Food
(TEF), 10%

Resting Metabolic Rate
(RMR), 60-75%%

The purpose of explaining metabolism in this much detail is to show how making small daily lifestyle changes using The PRISE Life and Protein Pacing Protocol can impact your overall metabolism and, more importantly, health and performance in major ways.

THE DIFFERENCE BETWEEN MEN AND WOMEN

Males typically have a higher RMR than females because they generally have a greater percentage of lean body mass than females of the same age. But don't let that deter you if you are a woman reading this book. The great news is that my research shows incredible weight loss results for both men and women who followed The PRISE Life Protocol, and neither group felt hungry! That alone is a win for this lifestyle program!

So, although it is true that women tend to have lower levels of lean muscle mass and a higher proportion of fat cells, and it is true that fat cells have a lower metabolic rate than lean muscle mass cells, I am telling you with total confidence, and scientific proof, that a healthy weight and body composition can still be attained no matter your chromosomes!

CAFFEINE AND METABOLISM

Over the years, I've studied many environmental and lifestyle factors that impact our metabolism, and one of the most powerful agents is caffeine. It's the most widely consumed drug in the world, and the intake of caffeine continues to grow in popularity. What's so fascinating is that caffeine has powerful effects on both our central (brain) and peripheral (muscles, fat, vital organs, etc.) nervous systems, so the magnitude of its effect is vast.

On top of that, caffeine is capable of both direct and indirect effects on the body. What this means is that caffeine has direct entry into the cells to exert an effect, and it can influence the levels of other substances (hormones, enzymes, etc.) in an indirect effect. So, given its widespread impact on our body, I conducted two large-scale, intensive research studies examining the metabolic, cardiovascular, and emotional/mood effects of caffeine in both women and men of varying ages. My findings were so impressive, *The Wall Street Journal*, *Men's Journal*, and other media outlets highlighted them.

WOMEN, MEN AND CAFFEINE

In both younger and older women, caffeine drastically increases the number of calories burned at rest; I call this the thermic response to caffeine. But older women burn half as many calories as younger women, and the amount of fat (fatty acids) appearing in the bloodstream (with the potential to be burned as energy) is similar between the younger and older women—this is great news! Interestingly, the thermic response to caffeine is positively associated with body weight and waist circumference in younger women, whereas positively related to aerobic fitness in older women. This means caffeine's effects may largely depend on body weight and waist size in younger women, but older women should remain active to get the biggest caffeine boost!

In terms of heart health, mood state, and caffeine in women, blood pressure is increased and feelings of depression are decreased in older women following caffeine intake. In younger women, some interesting findings occurred. For one, feelings of tension and vigor increased, and feelings of fatigue decreased. Second, those who are less physically active are more vulnerable to the blood-pressure-raising effects of caffeine than more active, younger women. (*It should be noted that these findings are limited to moderate consumers of caffeine who abstained for forty-eight hours prior to testing, and who ingested the equivalent of about two to three cups of caffeine, or 240 mg*).

Now for us guys. We respond differently to caffeine than women do. Both younger and older men show a similar thermogenic response to caffeine ingestion, but younger men release many more fatty acids into the bloodstream compared to older men following caffeine ingestion—this is not so great news for older men. Similar to women, older men increased blood pressure after caffeine ingestion, but younger men had no change. The mood state changes were fascinating; older men reduced feelings of tension and anger, whereas the younger guys reported feeling angrier ... uh, oh—you young guys need to watch your caffeine intake!

CHANGING METABOLISM WITH EXERCISE AND EATING

As a scientist, once we have determined the starting point of the individual's RMR—remember energy expended at rest—we then move into what happens when we add other lifestyle choices, such as caffeine, food, and exercise, to the process. The incredible fact about the body is that there are longer-term effects of frequent physical exercise, and they are that you can actually change the RMR. Some scientists have shown an increase in RMR, and others a decrease in RMR, with exercise training. The reason for this discrepancy is likely due to the level of fitness of the person. For example, highly trained elite athletes may show a decrease in RMR with intense training due to the metabolism slowing down and working more efficiently to conserve calories for when they are needed the most, which is during their intense training and competition.

Some scientists, myself included, have shown RMR to increase with exercise training. That is great news because once you have created a base calorie level and released the toxins, should you add exercise, you have the chance to consume higher quantities of healthy foods. You read that right! You will be able to eat more! Just in case that is not enough good news, the topper from some of my research is that even those participants who did not exercise, still lost significant weight!

THE METABOLIC TAKEAWAY

The secret? The entire weight-loss success was because of eating the right quality and amount of protein at the right time. This is the Protein Pacing discovery! Now you will have an entirely new interest in learning the value of protein, when to use it, and how much. And now that you understand metabolism and RMR, we can move on to learn about the different rates at which your body burns macronutrients (proteins, fats, and carbs). You won't have to spend another minute figuring this out for yourself! I'm excited knowing that you are getting a unique, science-based, truthful education, and that you care enough about yourself to keep plugging away! See, champion!

CHAPTER 11

THE MIRACLES OF MACROS: PROTEINS, FATS AND CARBS

What's behind you doesn't matter.
— Enzo Ferrari

In the last chapter, we reviewed the incredible biochemical process called human metabolism and that, simply, its job is to convert food into energy so your body can function. Now, we are going to dig a little deeper and talk about the next miracles.

Often the easiest way to understand the topic of macronutrients, and how each benefit our system, is to think of a race car. Again, we don't put diesel (or sugar) in a gas engine because it kills it. Putting unhealthy, processed, and prepackaged food into your body, as a staple, will eventually kill you too. So, pull in your imaginary dreaming brain and picture your body as a Ferrari, Maserati, Porsche, or Tesla (or that favorite car you dream of owning). I'm dreaming right along with you! Now, imagine how you would treat this dream car. I want you to commit to treating yourself better than your favorite car, starting today!

How exactly do you do that? That is what this chapter is all about.

MACRONUTRIENTS

Macronutrients are proteins, fats, and carbs, and they are the fuel that feeds us. However, like all fuels, the quality and quantity, the timing and the amount, all count. The human body is created perfectly, and each macronutrient has a valuable role to play. Macronutrients contained within food provide us energy and fuel. Once the food has been digested and is ready for absorption, transport, and entry into the cells of the body, we need to package these macronutrients into smaller units. Most of the carbs we eat become monosaccharides, the most abundant of which is glucose; fats or lipids become free fatty acids, while proteins become amino acids.

MACRO #1: PROTEIN

Let's start with protein because that is the key to Protein Pacing. The term protein originates from the Greek word proteios, meaning "primary," or "first," and is vital to human life. Protein is the major building block in the body, and it builds muscle, connective tissues, enzymes, immune cells, and is vital in so many cell-building roles. Even skin is built of protein. It is the most thermogenic, energy-costly (in a good way) nutrient we can eat.

What do I mean by energy costly? The beauty of protein is that it takes the body a lot of its own energy to digest, absorb, transport and metabolize it through an "active" process. Meaning, it requires a lot of energy to process and also triggers certain substances and hormones in the gut to be released and sent to the brain. This is why protein makes the body feel fuller longer than a carbohydrate. The process of using protein properly, in the right amount and at the right time, is the key to Protein Pacing. It is the best strategy to follow to help with weight wellness and peak performance, leading to ideal body composition, especially compared to carbohydrate, and even fat, overconsumption.

THE BUILDING BLOCKS OF PROTEIN: AMINO ACIDS

The building blocks of protein—amino acids—circulate in your bloodstream, portal circulation (liver), lymph system and make up the metabolic amino acid pool. The protein foods we eat have various fates inside the body, with almost 40% of the protein being catabolized (broken down) and even excreted, and only about 10% of the protein we eat is used by the muscles for protein synthesis and building of new muscle. Proteins are constantly broken down and the component parts used again and again, which is also why it's so important to protein pace to replenish the amino acids. This turnover rate is variable; some cells in your digestive system turn over in three to four days, while cartilage cells take years to turn over. This variability is important, because major organs like the liver, brain, and heart will be spared from breakdown during starvation at the expense of not-as-essential cells.

Protein is composed of twenty amino acids, and the great news is, if you consume the right amount at the right time, it will help you build healthy, calorie-burning lean muscle mass and keep your metabolism at a healthy level, which in turn will help you break down and release fat. Protein is essential to create lean muscle mass and repair tissues. When protein breaks down into the nine essential and eleven nonessential amino acids, it is doing so to keep you healthy and extend your life!

We know, from very good scientific investigations, that our bodies are ideally designed to absorb between 20–40g of protein per serving. How can you achieve this? Protein Pacing! The way to get the ideal amount of protein for optimal absorption by the gut and to maximally stimulate protein synthesis, is through Protein Pacing.

ESSENTIAL AND NONESSENTIAL AMINO ACIDS

It is fascinating to understand the difference between essential and nonessential amino acids, and believe it or not, this is where the right type of food is essential. The only way the body can get the nine essential amino acids (technically, eight for adults) to live is by the food we put in our mouths!

Understand how significant this is because you can either build up and support your body with proper use of good protein or you can destroy your body by leaving out some of the essential amino acids. We control this, no one else can, and we must, in essence, treat it like our favorite car! Therefore, while the nonessential amino acids simply mean that the body has a way of creating these internally, it is not quite as important that you get each of them in your body through food. However, it is important that you are eating the right sources of food to aid the overall process.

As for storing, it's well-known that protein, as a macronutrient, is not readily stored in the body as an energy source. Instead, the building blocks of protein, called amino acids, are used for nearly every cell of the body to help build new structures. For example, protein is the major supplier of tissue construction in our muscles, due to its structural function. On a per-volume basis, the brain is actually the largest consumer, or user, of amino acids.

Ultimately, Mother Hen, the liver, stores the greatest amount of amino acids as it gets ready to send them to the tissues that need to be repaired, rebuilt, or built new. But since muscle is the primary site for amino acid uptake to support muscle-cell growth, this is the way that bodybuilders to fitness and performance achievers use protein to build lean muscle mass and also amp up their RMR. Protein truly is the primary nutrient for our body.

PROTEINS ARE THE FRAME

Think about proteins as the entire exterior and interior frame of a car, including the wheels, and everything under the hood, like the engine (your heart is a muscle too!)

Remember, you only get one car body (including engine) for one lifetime. How are you going to treat it? Only you can keep it from rusting, getting flat tires, and breaking down year after year, and those nine essential amino acids that you make sure you get from the food will determine the longevity of the vehicle. Perhaps that will make you think twice about what is going into that body of yours!

MISCONCEPTIONS ABOUT PROTEIN

Thanks to the media, your fear when I tell you to eat protein, and fat, may be: "Oh, no, now I am definitely going to gain weight!" Not true. It is nearly impossible to gain fat from eating too much protein—one of the most well-known untruths in nutrition.

Of all the nutrients, protein in excess is the least likely to be converted to fat. In fact, in our current society, our intake of protein has declined in direct linear proportion to the increase in obesity since the 1970s. And, of all the macros, protein is the least likely to be used by the body to make energy. Its priority is to help build and repair cells and tissue. This is also a major reason why protein is not used and stored as an energy source (with the exception of small amounts of branched chain amino acids during stress, intense exercise, and prolonged starvation). They are too committed to the vital role of building and repairing tissues and cells.

And while we are talking about misconceptions, some people still believe that protein can only be found in meat and dairy products. This is far from the truth, because there are both animal and plant protein sources, and this opens up a whole new way of eating while getting healthy proteins into your body.

THE HIGH-PROTEIN DIET MISCONCEPTION

Thirty years of nutrition and metabolism research has taught me a valuable lesson: Our bodies thrive on a diet consisting of 25%-35% lean, healthy protein (from both plant and animal sources), along with at least 25% healthy fats and oils, lots of fresh veggies, certain whole grains, and fruit. Yet, even with scientific proof, there are still some non-believers.

Despite my published research, as well as research by others that supports a Protein Pacing plan, a recent article in the *New York Times*, "The Myth of High-Protein Diets," written by a well-known cardiologist (Dean Ornish, MD) cites a limited perspective of current dietary intake trends and the obesity epidemic using data from the US Department of Agriculture from 1950 to 2000.

In stark contrast, more recent peer-reviewed scientific data paints a much different picture of food-intake trends and prevalence of obesity among Americans from the period 1970–2010. While both sets of data agree that food intake increased about 200 calories per day during this time period, the source of where those additional calories came from differs drastically. Ornish places the blame on fat and protein. But the published data clearly shows Americans ballooned after eating too many of the wrong carbohydrates during this time period. In fact, current research data strongly supports that for every 1% increase in calories from protein and 1% reduction in carbohydrate calories, overall food intake may decrease by 33 calories a day! In other words, the more protein you eat, the less total calories you consume, and the more likely you will lose weight and improve your health.

PROTEIN HOLDS THE KEY TO WEIGHT LOSS

Protein (and fiber) holds the key to weight loss. Protein is a valuable nutrient for our bodies to help with healthy weight control and lean muscle mass. Protein is our metabolism's friend because it burns the most calories to digest compared to fat and carbohydrates. Let's look at each macronutrient a little closer. Several recent intervention studies from our laboratory provide strong support for eating a Protein Pacing diet—think a quarter to a third of your daily calories to decrease total body weight and body fat (including abdominal fat), while improving cardiovascular and metabolic health. Our study diets range between 25% and 35% high-quality animal and plant-based protein that emphasize foods such as nuts/seeds, legumes, beans, pea/rice protein powder, free-range eggs, grass-fed dairy products (milk, Greek yogurt, cottage cheese, whey protein powder), wild fish, and grass-fed beef.

In a lab, this can be easy to control, but from a practical standpoint, relying on only plants to meet your daily protein requirement can become a full-time job. For example, sound science has proven that four or more protein meals per day containing a minimum of 20g of protein optimizes protein synthesis, quenches hunger, and stimulates metabolism in people under sixty years of age, all of which help maintain the ideal body composition. Relying on only plant-based foods to meet this translates to 3½–5½ cups of cooked spinach, 1–2 cups of cooked lentils, or 2½–4½ cups of quinoa per meal. If you add physical activity and exercise to the mix, or age of sixty and older, you would require even more (up to 40g of protein per meal).

MEAT: THE VITAL PROTEIN

Meat is a vital protein source, and one that should be embraced. The important thing is to shop for meat with the same care many people put into shopping for vegetables: with a focus on quality. Not all animal meat is created equal. It is pretty well-known that differences exist between the quality of animal protein from conventional production facilities where the animals have been grain-fed in feedlots or cages versus free-roaming and pasture/grass-fed. Grass-fed beef has a greater amount of heart-healthy omega 3 fatty acids. This is the case for most animal protein sources, including milk, eggs, pork, and fish. Humanely treated and "in-the-wild" animal sources provide a healthier source of nourishment. This quality of animal protein also supports local farmers, which is great for the community and the environment.

So, I say, get your protein and don't be afraid of it. To summarize, I strongly recommend 25%-35% lean, healthy protein (from both plant and animal sources). Again, think protein as the car body; you only get one in a lifetime. What are you going to do to protect it like you would your favorite car?

MACRO #2: FATS

Continuing with the model of our body as a car, fats are the oil that feeds the rest of the engine. Just like a car needs oil, our bodies need oil (fats), high-quality oil to function. No matter how good the frame (protein) is, without oil, our engine will not work.

While fats take the longest time to generate ATP (energy) in the body, once they are broken down, they provide us with twice as much energy as either carbs or protein (9 versus 4 calories per gram). Fats are a highly efficient form of energy because they are stored without much, if any, water, and the body has nearly a limitless storage capacity of fat.

Now, what about the media hype that fat is what makes you fat? Let me clear that up, just like I cleared up that too much protein won't make you fat. Fat has had a terrible rap over the years with the low-fat craze, but please understand that your body needs fat, through good food choices, to protect and nourish vital organs like your heart and brain, and it is also essential in the assimilation of certain vitamins.

Fats provide us with lots of great benefits, such as insulation, energy, protection, hormone production, immune system support, etc. Because we store fats so readily in our bodies, the primary goal is to burn them for fuel every chance we get, especially at rest, while we sleep, and even during physical activity.

THE DANGERS OF STORED FAT

Before we look at how to use the macro called fat, let's take a moment to look at the dangers of building up fat. As a Fellow of the Obesity Society, we continue to monitor research and information, and the sad fact is that as a nation, the number of people struggling from obesity is increasing at an alarming rate.

The human body is designed to store fat relatively easy, and one way this happens is when we overeat carbs, especially simple carbs. As stated, the most popular sites for fat accumulation are under our skin (subcutaneous fat) and especially around the belly (abdominal fat) and our vital organs (visceral fat)—which is the most harmful. We also deposit fat and cholesterol inside our organs, which is definitely not good because it blocks blood and oxygen flow to vital organs such as the heart and brain.

People need to understand that we store fat in our cells and even carry them in the blood in the form of triglycerides. We are all well aware of how much fat we carry on our bodies, with most men storing it in their bellies and women around the hips and thighs—until menopause, when they also store it in the belly region. But what you might not know is that we also store a large proportion of fat inside our muscles and especially around our internal organs (visceral). It's this internal visceral fat that is the most dangerous, and increases our risk for cardiovascular (heart) and metabolic (diabetes) disease and certain cancers.

Much of my research has directly quantified/measured the amounts of the harmful visceral fat before and after following my prescribed nutrition and exercise program; the results have been astounding! Visceral fat is reduced by huge amounts every time. This is not a common occurrence with many weight loss and gimmick diets, so be careful. Calorie-restricting diets often cause weight loss in the form of subcutaneous fat loss and even muscle mass loss without a substantial amount of visceral fat; when this happens, it's disastrous! But you won't have to worry about this happening with my protocol. Much of the fat loss occurs in the belly and visceral fat region, and the proportion of lean muscle mass is preserved and even increases! Woo-hoo!

THE MISGUIDED LOW-FAT DIET

Fats have been ostracized and treated like the black sheep of the food group dating to the 1980 US Dietary Guidelines. In the early '80s, I vividly recall my dad trying to lose a few pounds and coming home from the grocery store each week with low/no-fat everything—ice cream, milk, cheese, cookies, crackers, yogurt, and even potato chips. Despite eating all of these low/no-fat foods, he struggled to lose those extra pounds. I think many people can relate here.

The most disturbing irony of the low/no-fat diet recommendation is that the more Americans have avoided eating fat, the fatter we've become as a nation. Yes ... the statistics are stunning, but there is much to learn from them.

Interestingly, the driving force behind the low/no-fat craze that swept the nation was the US Department of Agriculture (USDA) and the

Department of Health and Human Services (HHS). Up until recently, the group has emphasized low/no-fat foods.

It's pretty well-known that private interests and industry lobbyists played a major role in the misguided food-guide pyramids we've all been told to follow since 1980, and the low/no-fat recommendation was the first example of this. Fortunately, for the first time since 1980, the most current 2015 DGAC finally removed an upper limit on total fat intake. In other words, they lifted the ban on total fat intake and opened the door to accepting—even encouraging— dietary fat intake as a healthy part of the diet. The article cited here called "Lift the Ban on Total Dietary Fat," published by the *Journal of the American Medical Association* (JAMA), is worthy of a read. Progress!

EAT FAT TO BURN FAT

The scientific data is clear: We need to eat fat to burn fat and all fat is not the same. Even the *New York Times Magazine* in 2002 addressed this in an article called, "What If It's All Been a Big Fat Lie?" A diet rich in healthy fats, such as nuts and seeds (walnuts, almonds, macadamia, flax, chia), plant (olive, coconut, avocado, palm), and fish oils is the most nutritious and tasty.

Opting for the full-fat version of (organic and local) milk, cheese, Greek yogurt, and cage-free/free-range eggs is usually a better option than the low/no-fat versions; so don't be fooled. Keep in mind that fats/lipids are major components of every cell membrane in our body, and we have billions and billions of them. Fats regulate fluids that pass in and out of our cells, make cholesterol and hormones, and protect our nerve fibers—so never underestimate the role that they play.

THE IMPORTANCE OF CHOLESTEROL

We've heard so much about how bad cholesterol is for you that we tend to overlook its importance. It works right next to lipids in the cell membranes and makes the membranes rigid and able to hold their shape. There are many more membrane functions thought to be attributed to cholesterol's presence. Just like fat is used for insulation and shock absorption as it protects organs and joints from the trauma of movement, cholesterol is necessary for the body. Because we need it for health reasons, low-cholesterol diets are not necessarily good for us (unless you have a rare genetic variant that leads to excess plaque buildup, in which case you should aim to limit your intake to 200 mg/day).

In fact, dietary cholesterol from foods such as eggs (one egg yolk contains about 200mg) makes little impact on the cholesterol levels in your blood. Our daily requirement for cholesterol is about 300 mg/day. The less cholesterol you eat in foods, the more cholesterol your body produces itself. So, the amount of cholesterol you eat really only affects how much your body has to produce itself. Your liver (which I call Mother Hen) likes to keep the cholesterol to about 1,000 mg/day to support body needs.

Another extremely beneficial strategy to help lower total and LDL cholesterol (bad cholesterol) is with plant sterols from nuts, seeds, and legumes, as well as Pantethine, a derivative of vitamin B5 and niacin, B3. The sterols reduce the absorption of cholesterol by looking and acting just like cholesterol, and therefore block it from being absorbed by the gut and into the bloodstream. Aim to eat foods containing 1.3g of plant sterols a day.

BAD FATS VS. GOOD FATS

As I have stressed throughout the book, the quality of the fats is everything. To make it simple, don't eat trans fats. They are bad for you and are found in partially hydrogenated oils to make the substance more solid, like margarine or even shortening, and certain saturated fats (those that get hard at room temperature and come from conventional feedlot animal products), or vegetable shortenings—both increase blood cholesterol and are linked to heart disease.

The great news is, you don't have to be afraid of all fats. As a matter of fact, some are really good for you in the proper proportion. Included are monounsaturated fats like olive oil, which can even help lower blood cholesterol levels, and perhaps even polyunsaturated and saturated fats (the oils that come from the fish, plant, and vegetable origin and are liquid or soft at room temperature).

The most important fact to walk away with is that good fats don't make you fat; they can even lower blood cholesterol levels and help you maintain energy and proper weight. So, please, take another look at fats in foods and do choose to incorporate the healthy ones! I recommend at least 25% healthy fats and oils and up to as much as 70% if you are following the fat-adapted, ketogenic diet.

MACRO #3: CARBS

Finally, we arrive at the truth about those carbs! Carbohydrates can't be ignored. Sticking with the car analogy, carbs are your fuel or gas! Put in cheap, leaded up gas and your car is going to spit and sputter along … put in high octane, lead-free gas and your car is going to burn some rubber! Every part of metabolism has been put in order by the creator for a reason. If you have been part of the no-carb phase, I want you to rethink things a little bit. I want to help you realize why you may be so tired. The wrong carbs, or no carbs to give you quick energy, are probably weighing you down, and therefore, you are resorting to caffeine or other sources of stimulants to try to get through the day.

The fact is, the right carbohydrates truly are the main, and first, energy sources for the brain and red blood cells throughout the day. Carbs break down into glucose. You need glucose for the brain to function and for your muscles to function efficiently during the day, and especially while exercising.

Unfortunately, given our excessively high intake of carbohydrates in our culture on a daily basis, especially simple sugars, we accumulate and store a lot of excess fat from overeating simple carbs, much more so than an excess intake of fat or protein.

Just to be clear, simple carbs are those that are digested quickly, such as the sugar in soda and candy, fruit juices, but also the refined and processed cakes, bread, and pasta. Complex carbs that include fiber digest more slowly, don't play havoc with your blood sugar, and are much more advisable.

DEBUNKING THE CARB MYTHS

And now for the fun, debunking part, as I talk about "wonder carbs," and I don't mean Wonder Bread! In recent years, no single food group has been thrown under the bus more than carbohydrates. This carb backlash reminds me of the low-fat craze I discussed. I want to remove the diet clutter and nutrition misinformation and set the record straight on both fat and carbohydrate intake.

Perhaps you're gluten-sensitive, have celiac disease, or you're boycotting all GMO carbs. I get it … these are all valid and real reasons to keep an eye on your carb intake and not overindulge. However, none of these are healthy and safe excuses to avoid carbs completely. Carbohydrates come in many different forms, including vegetables, fruits, legumes (beans and nuts), whole grains, and even dairy. To suggest that a no-carb diet is remotely safe and healthy is dangerous. Our bodies need carbs because they provide energy, healthy fiber and essential nutrients, boost immunity, and give food sweetness.

The biggest challenge is choosing carb foods that provide the most nourishment and health benefits, yet also taste good. We love our bread, bagels, pasta, potatoes, rice, and cookies, but these are the main culprits to storing excess body fat, especially belly fat. We all know the benefits of eating fresh vegetables and fruits and the health problems of too many starchy carbs.

HOW THE BODY PROCESSES MACROS

To lose fat, the fat molecule needs oxygen and a background level of carbohydrates to complete the chemical breakdown. It is important to ensure your body has an adequate supply of high-quality carbohydrates. When this carb supply is exhausted, the body struggles in burning fat the way it usually does and instead starts to break down fat in a process called ketosis.

Our goal should always be to preserve our muscle mass because muscles provide definition and tone. It's also a source of fat-burning, since it burns more calories than fat. There is a huge advantage to getting fit so your body can become a fat-burning machine, both at rest and during submaximal exercise.

QUALITY, OVER QUANTITY

It is less about the quantity of food you're eating than it is the quality of food that you are ingesting! For the record, I never mention weight loss or dieting to my clients, athletes, and research study participants. I am not concerned whether they lose any weight at all, and I do not focus on *how many calories* they are eating or burning with exercise. I avoid a *calorie-*

counting mentality and instead encourage nourishment through eating the right types of food and choosing the right types of exercise and activity.

If you are nourishing your body throughout the day with the right type, amount, and timing of the most critical and vital nutrients your body needs to function optimally—with the right amount of protein to keep your muscles and cells functioning optimally and signal to the brain that it's satisfying—you will maximize your health and performance and have the energy to add fitness training. I fully understand and appreciate the laws of thermodynamics when it comes to calories in and calories out, but lots of really good science supports the major role of protein tipping the scale as a superior macro to support optimal body weight and composition.

I am all about helping people optimize their overall health, body composition, and physical performance by teaching and guiding them with scientifically proven lifestyle strategies to achieve their best results and keep them motivated and committed to staying on a healthy path.

When you follow The PRISE Life Protocol, you will have the best side effect ever! You will find it to be an effective strategy to accelerate body fat (especially belly fat) loss; build lean muscle mass; enhance metabolism; lower blood sugar, cholesterol, and blood pressure; release toxins from body fat, and greatly enhance physical performance. By following a healthy lifestyle program such as PRISE—that incorporates scientifically proven strategies that show you how to eat healthier, exercise properly, and reduce stress—you will not have to worry.

With our little refresher course on macronutrients, understanding quality over quantity, not counting calories, you are now primed to understand how important each macronutrient is and a little about their true roles. In the end, metabolism and getting the proper macronutrients are all about energy expenditure to give your body life power, and by balancing it is revealing the correct amounts to use when, so you, too, can gain optimal health.

Overall, human nutrition and metabolism are evolving so rapidly that it's important to have access to the latest scientific research on the health and performance benefits of all different types of food, including proteins, fats, and carbs, as well as immediately dispelling the new myths that seem to be spreading rapidly every day.

I hope this also helps you understand why my research has been validated and embraced worldwide. I don't want you to have a shortened "shelf life" because you ignored the natural life cycles of our food and our bodies, or you didn't pay attention to the value and purpose of macronutrients. I want you to live and eat and find the energy and life source that makes you abundant—that makes you a gift to the universe as you were meant to be. I want your Maserati or Porsche to last a long, long time.

KEY POINTS ON NUTRITION

- The longer-than-normal shelf life of many foods wreaks havoc on the human body because the harmful chemicals used to protect and stimulate the growth of the vegetable, fruit, grain, or animal gets passed on to the cells in our bodies.
- Synthetic chemicals contribute to the current plague of modern-day diseases, such as cardiovascular and metabolic disease, certain cancers, as well as inflammatory and neurodegenerative disorders.
- Macronutrients in the right portions at the right time, especially protein, will make almost any diet program you follow a success.

Once you start following The PRISE Life Protocol, your body will understand that it is healing. The conversations within your cells will multiply and even speed your healing and performance. The beautiful nourishment from the new food and nutrients you are giving it will produce more energy efficiency and, as a result, give you more strength, breathing power, and endurance—more life power to enjoy.

That is the power that Mother Nature gives to us.

Will you choose a life that will help others and yourself thrive and find balance or will you continue to destroy the gift of life you have been given? I am giving you the keys. The keys to your priceless car. I am unparalyzing you by providing up-to-date, time-tested material that has already been shared with millions and is having lifesaving effects. It is your turn to choose the most incredible life energy around!

CHAPTER 12

WHAT ARE YOU FEEDING YOUR MIND?

Champions aren't made in the gyms.
Champions are made from something they have
deep inside them—a desire, a dream, a vision.
— Muhammad Ali, legendary boxer

BE A CHAMPION!

What does it take to be a champion? As a successful athlete myself, I have first-hand knowledge of what it takes. As a tennis champion, a winning triathlete, road race competitor, snowshoeing gold medalist, and competitive hockey player, I know that it takes drive and a desire deep within. I know that to be a champion, we must have the right thoughts. As a scientist who studies human physiology, nutrition, and neuropsychology, I also know there are mysteries of the mind that go way beyond what numbers and statistics could ever tell us. As analytical as I am, I have a

181

deeper belief in spiritual concepts. I believe in using every power possible to gain the advantage.

Games can be won or lost in our minds well before we show up for a competition, and that is what this chapter is all about. This chapter is about mental fitness and how it can help you reach your peak fitness and physical-performance goals. I have all the tools you need, so I am hypnotizing, programing, and encouraging you with these very words— with the backing of the universe. Today is the day, with this book in hand, you will create a maintainable and healthy lifestyle that will help you achieve optimal health and fitness. Repeat after me. "Today is the day, with this book in hand, I will create a maintainable and healthy lifestyle that will help me achieve optimal health and fitness." Believe it.

I want you to reach down deep and start to really think about what you love, what you are afraid of, sports you've dreamed of trying but maybe you were too scared, things you want to achieve, and ways to remove all the obstacles. I want you to know that optimal health is in your future. I have created something for everyone. You have that champion in you; you only have to decide and then go find him or her.

THE POWER OF OUR THOUGHTS

The Abraham-Hicks laws of attraction teach that you create your world with every thought. This is a powerful tool for transformation through nutrition and fitness. Metabolism is really an energy and vibrational response at any moment in time inside our body. As such, many believe this energy determines everything about us, including our thoughts and feelings, and therefore it is truly mind (energy) over matter. If we accept that we have a deep influence over what happens to our metabolism, as we also have over what happens to our health, fitness, and wellness, then all the more reason we need to be careful what we think, and especially what we say.

We also need to seriously consider who we keep around us, because negative people breed negative energy, and there is no time for your metabolism, your mind, or your body to pick up any of those sensations from those with limited-thinking or those who are uninformed. Surround yourself with those who love you unconditionally, and learn to love yourself as you are at this moment, knowing that very soon you will be the best-ever you. In fact, new research out of Harvard University finds that happiness is truly contagious, but so are obesity and smoking! So choose your company wisely! This will support the lifestyle changes of The PRISE Life.

The mental side of optimal health and peak performance is just as important as the physical side, because not only does it help you develop deep spiritual commitments that tune you up for success, but it also helps you become aware of what your body is saying to you. Your mind can help you find nutrient-dense, high-quality foods more attractive, it can nudge you when you are down and show you the value of mood-enhancing endorphins when you exercise, and it will even tell you when today is a day for rest.

EXCELLENCE

Vince Lombardi said, "Perfection isn't attainable, but if we chase perfection we can catch excellence." I believe that excellence comes with commitment and honesty and follow-through, even when you don't think you have an ounce of energy left to succeed. Excellence comes from creating a clean slate with a pure heart and simply accepting that past failures happened, but never letting them define or defeat you. Excellence is always putting your best foot forward, knowing that some days you will trip and end up with mud on your face, and excellence is always being loving, kind, and good to others, no matter how you may be feeling yourself.

In excellence, you start to choose healthy and nutritionally packed foods because they are our friends; food is our healer. It is how we say to our bodies, "I love you back." Your body is your temple. You need to treat it well, and it will reward you in return. This is what my research says! One of my studies examined the mood enhancement of Protein Pacing with and without physical exercise. It was real. It was definable and thereby is achievable for all of you.The bottom-line finding from my research shows that nourishing your body with Protein Pacing, including high-quality protein, fats and carbs, results in a better mood, and when you add fitness to the equation, the results look even more promising.

PACING IN ALL AREAS OF LIFE

We discussed the amazing benefits of Pacing with Protein in Chapter 3. But pacing is a concept that is important for every part of our being, including our relationships and our emotional/spiritual well-being. Science shows that the quality of our relationships is significantly enhanced when we take the time to be present with another person, even if it's only for a few minutes at a time. This is pacing.

Pacing is also important in our emotional and spiritual lives. As part of my PRISE Life Protocol, I've included a "body visit," which is a daily mindfulness-awareness meditation that includes a breathing exercise and time spent in quiet reflection. Visualize daily having a long and healthy life, and the laws of attraction will bring that energy your way. Again, pacing is what's important to maximize the benefit.

TRAIN HARD, BELIEVE HARDER

Life energy is power that is ignited by metabolism in the body, and is sparked by a thought in the mind. It creates you. It motivates you. It is what inspires you. If you have ever been coached or involved in a team sport, you will have been taught strategies to help you get over losses or challenges. The most important strategy is to train hard (healthy-hard as you learned in Part 1), but BELIEVE even harder.

This is about enjoying your life along the way and working steadily to achieve your health, fitness, and performance goals. And your beliefs, especially about your body, make all the difference. It's not how fast you start but how long you last. Balance.

HEALTHY CHOICES AND SELF-CARE

You can be well if you choose to. For example, do we make the choice to eat a healthy snack, such as a banana with peanut butter or carrots and hummus, or do we choose instead to eat a donut or bagel with cream cheese? Do we choose to stand up from our chair every hour and take a brisk five-to-ten-minute walk around the house or office? These are all healthy choices that you can make: standing up at your computer, walking around, stepping outside, doing some qi gong, putting your bare feet on the ground.

The starting point of any new healthy lifestyle lies in our heads. It means self-care. The best health care is self-care. The best self-care is the food we eat, the exercise we do, and the spiritual mindfulness we practice. That's why I developed The PRISE Protocol. Self-care, because it suggests the greatest resource to improve our health, resides within each of us. Have you heard the saying, "Physician, heal thyself"?

Why is it important to choose to be well in the first place? Of course, there are the obvious and well-known health reasons such as a reduced risk for obesity, heart disease, diabetes, cancer, cognitive decline, and mental illness, among others. Perhaps even more powerful are the subjective reasons, including clearer thinking, enhanced mental and emotional well being, greater productivity at work and home, and more physical energy to spend time playing with kids, grandkids, and loved ones.

We need to take charge of our minds, get our heads in the game, and think about what we may be doing to sabotage ourselves. After all, what excuse do we really have not to get well?

OVERCOMING OBSTACLES STARTS IN THE MIND

I know there are many obstacles out there. I have been knocked down my fair share of times. For example, how do you exercise when you work eighteen hours a day, or when you have no energy? Obstacles are going to be there every day, but you don't have to bring energy to them. You start with your mind and thinking positive thoughts.

You are a winner despite, or better yet, because of all your failures, and right now you are going to absolutely let go of negative thinking or comparing yourself to others. Those emotions and thoughts bring your body down and confuse your cells. You will be amazed how the minute you change your thoughts, any imagined lack will disappear from your life and abundance and gratitude will fill in that space.

MY MANTRA: "KEEP YOUR EYES ON THE PRISE!"

When we face obstacles, it is helpful to have a mantra that we can repeat to get us through! Years ago, when I created my protocol, this mantra came to me and has always stuck. It is the title of a song by folk singer Pete Seeger: "Keep Your Eyes on the Prize." He made sure to introduce gospel songs as he traveled the world sharing his *We Shall Overcome* album. His purpose was to share the power of words.

There is power in words, there is power in intention. The true origin of the song is given to English Folk Songs from the Southern Appalachians, published in 1917. Many gospel songs were based on pulling in strength from God. They were created, and sung, as rhythmic chants to keep one's mind and focus on something else. In times of deep suffering, abuse, poverty, and cruelty, many had to turn to a Higher Power to get through, to survive. I share the words of this song here so that they might inspire you when you need some motivation:

Paul and Silas bound in jail
Had no money for to go their bail
Keep your eyes on the prize, hold on

Paul and Silas thought they were lost
Dungeon shook and the chains come off
Keep your eyes on the prize, hold on

Freedom's name is mighty sweet
And soon we're gonna meet
Keep your eyes on the prize, hold on

I got my hand on the gospel plow
Won't take anything for my journey now
Keep your eyes on the prize, hold on

Only chain that a man can stand
Is that chain o' hand on hand
Keep your eyes on the prize, hold on

I'm gonna board that big greyhound
Carry the love from town to town
Keep your eyes on the prize, hold on

Now the only thing I did was wrong

Stayin' in the wilderness too long
Keep your eyes on the prize, hold on

The only thing we did was right
Was the day we started to fight
Keep your eyes on the prize, hold on

Hold on, hold on
Keep your eyes on the prize, hold on

Ain't been to heaven but I been told
Streets up there are paved with gold
Keep your eyes on the prize ... hold on!

The inspiration for this song comes from Acts 16:19–26 in the Bible, about Paul and Silas, both Jews, who were marched through town and thrown in jail for not following the Roman customs of the day. They were beaten, starved, stripped naked, and shackled. There was no way out, and nothing was going to save them. Until ... They started singing hymns that praised God. Incredible! Envision that you are in the deepest, darkest time of your life, and instead of lashing out in anger, hurt, and fear, you start singing praises to the Creator. That's pretty impressive in my view!

I've been in those moments where there was nothing left to do but cry out for clarity and help, and the mantra from this song has helped me so much! I hope it will help you too, when you face obstacles in your quest for optimum health. So, "Keep Your Eyes on the PRISE!" Hold on, hold on, because I have a scientifically proven roadmap to take you on.

WHAT IS YOUR INSPIRATION?

In addition to having a mantra, we all need a source of inspiration to help us when we face challenges—a story that puts our lives into perspective and helps us to choose health and wellness. Let me share mine.

It was a cold, wintry morning in 1983 in Connecticut. I was in my junior year in college and I was working as a fitness instructor. My supervisor asked me to train a young woman. As an exercise science major in college and an athlete, I thought I was prepared for just about anyone who walked into the gym. But I was not prepared for Tina, who was pushed into the gym in her wheelchair. She had cerebral palsy, and at nineteen, was the same age as I was at the time.

For the next hour, I led Tina through an exercise program with the help of my supervisor. Tina, in her compromised physical condition, pushed herself to her limit and seemingly enjoyed the workout with me. I was transformed—my spark was lit. I still remember sitting in my cold car in the gym parking lot for several long minutes that day reflecting on how powerful an experience it was to witness first-hand. As my eyes welled up with tears, all I could think about was how strong her resolve and desire was "to be well" and healthy.

In fact, it was right then and there, in my cold, beat-up fifteen-year-old car that I decided to devote my life to help others experience the same opportunity to be well that I shared with Tina on that blustery, cold day. In truth, it was a life-changing epiphany and made me realize that sharing health and wellness with others is contagious, and it's a two-way street. I learned just as much, if not more, about being well and healthy from Tina as she learned from me that day. I continue to learn and grow from the many students, athletes, research-study participants, and clients that I work with on how to achieve optimal health and wellness.

What is your inspiration to keep going when things get hard? Find something, or someone, that reminds you: Drop the excuses, you CAN do this! There is someone you know who is overcoming insurmountable problems and probably hasn't ever complained! Every day I try to choose to be well so that I can give back to others more fully, the same way Tina gave to me.

OUR MENTAL CONDITIONING

Recently, I came upon a program called Quantum Emergence that is all about discovering the triggers of our emotions and how the pain and suffering we experience in our lives have shaped us. We often refer to this as our "conditioning." If you are truly stuck, can't commit to a plan, can't get your head in the game, perhaps consider taking a look at your conditioning and beliefs and how they affect your emotions.

The strongest psychological human drive is to behave consistently with the belief we have about ourselves, which perpetuates the same old behaviors over and over again—mind you, not good behaviors! This drive is faulty and not accurate and is rooted in the subconscious that relies on early life experiences that originally caused those same emotions, feelings, and reactions.

It's in recognizing that early childhood forms the basis of our belief system and, more times than not, they are false and inaccurate. We must go more deeply into our life experiences and understand that once we can target, explore, and realize these original events, we can finally be allowed to overcome our obstacles and our emotions and move into our true being, identity, and calling. It is this truth that I want you to embrace so that you have a chance to succeed and prosper. You are valuable. Your life has meaning, and it is time to honor every part of you, releasing the old and embracing the new.

The clearer and more focused you can become, the more healthy and successful you will become. Your path seems to make more sense, and your direction and purpose become more clear. When you find that balance, something miraculous happens, something called second nature steps in!

SECOND NATURE

Second nature is being able to play the piano years after stopping, or being able to pick up a tennis racket after you haven't hit a ball in years and find that you can still rally the ball. All of those things are second nature. They are automatic and can save you when you have learned something the proper way, but second nature can also be harmful if it is a bad physical or emotional pattern that you have learned.

Second nature is one of the things top performers such as athletes, surgeons, actresses/actors, musicians, dancers, and top executives are coached on to become the best in their fields, leaders, and champions. My good friend refers to this as "mastering self-regulation." After you have carefully practiced a skill over and over and over until it has become second nature, you let go and let the body do the work without fighting it. Experts refer to this as "Mind 1" and "Mind 2." Mind 1 is the critic and judge and always analyzes everything we do, whereas Mind 2 just lets us be without any judging or criticizing. It's with Mind 2 that we can reach our full potential and achieve peak performance. It requires practice and determination to let healthy choices become second nature.

USING SPONTANEITY FOR PEAK PERFORMANCE

There is a fascinating book I've been reading titled *Trying Not to Try: The Art and Science of Spontaneity*, by Edward Slingerland. I am a true believer in hard work; however, as I get a little older and wiser, I am much more about working smarter! And no matter your age, it's better to learn this at an earlier stage, because it will help keep you from unnecessary strains, injuries, and overexertion on the body. In this book, Asian Studies professor Slingerland shares his concept of Wu-Wei (ooo-way) and DE (duh), which deals with spontaneity to foster peak performance.

Wu-Wei's message is really intriguing because it frees up our minds and allows us to achieve optimal health and peak performance without punishing our bodies by being held hostage and suffering. He teaches how to use spontaneity and effortless flow so exercise and performance can become natural without needing conscious thought. This is how the best performers operate at their peak of performance.

The exciting and amazing part is that this is exactly what I did when I created The PRISE Protocol. I made it easy to follow, easy to understand. I brought diversity to it so you never get bored, and I achieved my goal of making it second nature so that you don't have to think about it or use conscious thought and effortful striving, but instead follow the strategies by just doing.

To truly reach your peak, and stay there, it needs to become second nature to you and become a permanent lifestyle protocol. Because of this, I am all for discovering anything that may be holding you back and finding a good coach, physically or psychologically, to get you through if you need help.

TREAT YOURSELF LIKE A CHAMPION

Former NFL coach Jimmy Johnson said, "Treat a person as he is, and he will remain as he is. Treat him as he could be and he will become what he should be." I am telling you in no uncertain terms that you are a champion. You deserve champion treatment. It could be in your relationships, your work, your writings, your art, your athletic abilities, your Tai Chi, your yoga, I don't care what, but you have to believe, you have to know, you are the champion. You champion your body with your thoughts, and so today

I want you to give yourself a talk, a hug, some self-love, and tell yourself, and your soul, that regardless of what you see in the mirror, or in the blood tests, that these so-called facts do not control you. You control you.

You are the final champion, and you know you are the best. You will win every day you try. You will win every day you eat better. You will win every day you stand up and get outside in nature. You will win every day you set your mind right by getting rid of negative thoughts. You will win every day that your spirit is asked to help, and it picks you up off the floor of desperation to make it the best day of your life. Your heart will fill so full of gratitude, love for yourself, and others that success will be steps away, days away, not months, not years, but now.

And when, or if, you think you are having a bad day, know that you are my champion and that if you pull out the little statements and encouragements and truths in this book, they will pull you up and out to become the winner you deserve to be every . . . single . . . solitary moment of your life. So come on! Aren't you ready to follow every protocol in this book and to join me at the peak?

CHAPTER 13

TWO KEYS TO REJUVENATE YOUR BODY

*Sleep is that golden chain that ties
health and our bodies together.*
— *Thomas Dekker*

After I wrote this chapter, I seriously thought about moving it to the front of the book because I think it's that important. We live in a culture that considers rest, recovery, rejuvenation, and sleep as signs of being weak and not tough enough. Nothing could be further from the truth. In fact, if you consider the most successful people in the world from all different fields, they have one thing in common—extreme resilience. That's right, the ability to recover quickly from adversity or setback and come back even stronger. There is little question that the top performers in the world have enormous resilience that is built on a rock-solid foundation of rest, recovery, rejuvenation, and sleep! This chapter is about how important it is to restore and replenish your energy reserves, and that starts with sleep.

ARE YOU SLEEPING ENOUGH?

Ernest Hemingway once said, "I love sleep. My life has the tendency to fall apart when I'm awake, you know?" I am sure we can all relate to that some days! The truth is we need sleep, and many people underestimate the quantity and quality of their sleep. I routinely speak to audiences of all sizes, ages, and in all states of health, on a variety of health, wellness, and fitness topics. Every time I share the recommended goal of seven to eight hours of sleep per night for adults (and nine-plus hours for those under eighteen years old), I hear sighs, moans, and even chuckles.

In reality, most people fall well below these sleep recommendations, and for those close to meeting the recommendation, the quality (depth) of their sleep is often poor. Research studies consistently show that poor sleep quantity and quality are related to increased risk of conditions such as heart disease, high blood pressure, diabetes, obesity, depression, and stress, as well as decreased brain function (cognition). Sleep loss is also related to increased drug use among adolescents.

Lifestyle choices such as good nutrition, exercise, and mindfulness, etc. have a powerful impact on improving both sleep quality and quantity. In this chapter, I will share some of the important strategies for improving your health and well-being.

NUTRITION STRATEGIES FOR IMPROVING SLEEP

Trim the fat and sugar: In the Journal of Clinical Sleep Medicine, a group of researchers demonstrated that those with diets containing lower fiber and higher saturated fat and sugar have lighter, less restorative sleep and take a longer time to fall asleep and wake up more during the night.

The study showed that slow-wave sleep, which is the deepest, most restful, sleep, and the time needed to fall asleep were the most negatively impacted by a poor diet. So … reducing fat and sugar intake close to bedtime is a no-brainer. I strongly recommend a high-fiber and lean protein meal or snack one to two hours prior to your bedtime (BBB smoothie is ideal) to maximize sleep duration and depth.

Bean me up!   In a similar study called "Beans Improve Sleep," a group of scientists analyzed the diets and sleep patterns of more than a thousand adults. They found that the prevalence of adequate quantity and quality of sleep was not good (13% and 56%, respectively). The biggest finding was that optimal sleep duration and depth (quality) was greatest among those individuals with the highest intake of foods containing the plant chemicals known as isoflavones (daidzein genistein), found in soybeans, chickpeas, and other legumes. Other top nutrition choices to aid sleep:

> 4–8 oz. of tart cherry juice mixed with a small serving of your favorite plant or animal-based protein powder
>
> 4–7 oz. of pumpkin seeds
>
> 200mg of magnesium citrate
>
> 1-5mg of melatonin (optional)
>
> Avoid all caffeine after noon (especially if you are caffeine-sensitive or have trouble sleeping).

EXERCISE, ENVIRONMENT, AND SLEEP

Staying physically active is a natural sleep aid as well, but limit vigorous exercise for one to two hours before going to bed at night.

The benefits of napping have been known for a long time, and for good reason, especially following a sleep-deprived night. If you find yourself dozing off at your desk at work, steal away for a ten-to-twenty-minute nap.

Chances are, you will feel refreshed, mentally sharp, and ready to move your body.

Here are a few additional strategies to a better night's sleep:

- **Have regular sleep times:** Having a consistent bedtime is good for everyone, but a regular rise time, in the morning, is even more important for healthy sleeping.

- **Hibernate like a bear and create your own cave:** A dark, cool (58–64°F) room is best for deep sleep, just like hibernating animals. Try a sleeping mask if the room has too much natural light.

- **Avoid caffeine after breakfast:** Limit caffeine-containing foods and drinks after the morning meal.

- **Unplug:** Emerging research shows that the backlight from cellphones and other mobile devices (e-readers, laptops, etc.) remain illuminated inside the brain hours after you turn them off and affect your sleep quality and mood. So unplug at least two hours before you hit the pillow.

- **Body visit:** This is my go-to and I hope you make it yours (see the next section).

- **Fine-tune your sleep:** Avoid intense exercise in the evening; if you drink alcohol, do so in moderation; eat your dinner slowly, and minimize spicy and gassy foods.

THE BENEFITS OF BREATHING DEEPLY

Don't underestimate the value of just breathing. Deep-breathing techniques have existed and been used by yogis, and others, throughout the centuries. We are still learning the hidden values of paying attention to your breath. Shallow breathing is problematic, and for some reason, our bodies seem to resort to this when we are under stress or nervous. If we simply pay attention and take deep breaths, we would help ourselves tremendously. To be clear, the type of breathing I am talking about is inhaling deeply, and exhaling deeply! Don't hold your breath (whether in exercise or yoga). It is better when you breathe in a deep and rhythmic manner.

Deep breathing also helps accelerate metabolism because we are allowing more oxygen into the bloodstream. It helps your digestion to burn fat as fuel, and without enough oxygen, the food can't metabolize. Breathing brings in oxygen, which is crucial for all the systems of the body. Exhaling releases carbon dioxide and helps your body get rid of noxious gases and toxins.

MEDITATIVE BREATHING

I highly recommend diaphragmatic or belly breathing (sometimes called mindfulness breathing) throughout the day. Here's how it works:

- Close your eyes, or gaze gently five to seven feet in front of you.
- Begin by inhaling slowly using a five-second count.
- Hold your breath for two to three seconds.
- Exhale to a count of five.
- Repeat until you feel relaxed and peaceful.
- As you become more comfortable with this technique, extend the time for each phase to a seven-second inhale, five-second hold, and ten-second exhale.

THE IMPORTANCE OF MEDITATION

During those twelve years that my wife and I were completely maxed out on life, I suffered terribly from panic disorder. It became so overwhelming at times that I couldn't leave the house for days. I was in and out of doctors' offices for weeks at a time looking for them to solve my health problems. Instead of looking within to solve the root of my problem, I was stuck on looking for someone or something from the outside to fix me. I had it all wrong. Life was rough during this time.

Thankfully, with the help of my wife and family, and a continual dose of mind-body training and prayer, I was eventually able to pull myself out of this abyss. I have two "Emotional Nourishment" techniques that I want to share with you. I call them the "Body Visit" and "Mindfulness Awareness Meditation" (MAM). They provide the emotional nourishment we need to stay in balance and harmony, and to keep us moving and motivated. These bring all the forms of nourishment together to harmonize our bodies and fully integrate our minds, bodies, and spirits into one healthy human.

There are different ways to use these to attain emotional and spiritual fulfillment. I encourage you to use either of these meditations while doing other types of PRISE activities, such as stretching or endurance exercises.

THE BODY VISIT, PART 1

There are many different forms of meditation, but my favorite is fairly straightforward. When I was struggling to find emotional fulfillment in my own life, my oldest brother, John, taught me this Body Visit. You can do the Body Visit in one of three positions:

1) Sit in a chair, feet on the floor, back straight, arms relaxed by your side, hands resting on your lap.
2) Sit cross-legged on the floor on a comfortable cushion, arms resting on your thighs, palms facing the sky.
3) Lie on your back in the "savasana" position, legs spread apart, feet flopping to the side, with the flesh of your glutes pulled out from under you so the lower part of your spine is resting on the floor, arms extended away from your body, palms turned up to the sky with your shoulders relaxed away from your ears.

Putting lavender essential oil on the soles of your feet or burning a lavender candle may induce greater relaxation.

Start by taking several deep abdominal breaths. This is called diaphragmatic breathing, or belly breathing, or pranayama in yoga. Inhale down into the lowest part of your lungs, causing the abdomen (belly) to rise and fall on inhalation and exhalation. Research shows that this type of breathing reduces oxidative stress and increases antioxidant defense status in athletes.

Following three deep abdominal breaths, perform two more, but this time, as you inhale, close your eyelids and slowly roll your eyes counterclockwise (actually imagine turning back the clock of time!) by starting with your eyes staring downward and then slowly them until you are staring skyward, keeping your eyes closed the entire time. Try to keep your inhalation to five seconds. When you reach the end of inhalation, hold for three seconds with your eyes looking upward. Start your exhalation and continue rolling your eyes in the same counterclockwise direction, arriving back to where you started with your eyes gently gazing downward.

The exhalation should be seven seconds. Perform this two times and try pausing for four second between your inhalation and exhalation. With each breath, feel the new air reaching down to your toes and fingertips. Begin to release any tension you are feeling.

Continue to breathe in a relaxed, deep, and consistent manner as you feel your body letting go of all tension with each exhalation. During each inhalation, feel fresh, new, and revitalizing air circulating throughout your body.

Once you feel connected to your breath, you can move on to another common form of meditation referred to as contraction-relaxation meditation.

CONTRACTION-RELAXATION MEDITATION

Starting with your forehead, eyes, cheeks, lips, and other muscles of your face, along with your neck muscles, forcefully contract/tense all of them for two to four seconds. Then, let your face completely relax by having your eyelids fall over your eyes and allowing your mouth to hang open. Feel your ears begin to relax to the ground.

Next, tighten all the muscles in your shoulders, upper back, arms, and hands by clenching your fists and shrugging your arms and shoulders up to your ears and hold for two to four seconds, then exhale and completely relax all of these muscles. Allow your hands to open to the sky and your shoulder blades to sink to the ground. Imagine all the muscles of your arms completely melting to the ground and becoming very heavy.

Continue this same process with your abdomen, hips, thighs, gluteals, legs, calves, and feet until you've contracted and relaxed all the muscles in your body so you are fully aware of how you are feeling.

Once you've completed both the belly breathing and the contraction-relaxation meditation, begin to feel the tension disappear from your forehand, eyes, mouth, cheeks, and neck muscles. Allow your mouth to hang open and the small of your neck begins to soften and sink to the ground. Allow your ears to relax and all the muscles of your face to sink to the ground.

Next, bring your attention to your shoulders, arms, and hands. Release the tension between your shoulder blades by pulling your shoulders and arms away from your spine to create more space between your shoulder blades. Again, feel your belly rising with each breath in and falling with each breath out. Your exhalation should last longer than your inhalation and provide you with a feeling of deeper relaxation. Finally, feel the muscles of your hips, thighs, calves, and feet begin to relax and sink down away from your bones so they feel heavy and loose. You are now ready to begin your journey into the Body Visit mindfulness-awareness meditation.

THE BODY VISIT, PART 2

With your body in a new state of relaxation, allow any thoughts entering your mind to pass by without holding any judgment to them. Imagine each thought as raindrops hitting your car windshield and the wipers clearing them away so that none of them stay very long but instead get wiped away with each passing of the wiper blade. Another way to release your thoughts is to imagine them scrolling by as a ticker-tape passes highlights of news events at the bottom of your TV screen; none of them stay longer than a few seconds.

The true value of the Body Visit is that it allows you to move from a state of human nature (also known as subconscious) into a state of higher nature, or superconscious. This allows us to drop into the "flow state," a higher level of living and experiencing life. The flow state allows us to be in a higher nature and live to our full potential with creativity, problem-solving, and freedom.

GUIDED BODY VISIT WITH IMAGERY

One strategy that I've used since I was a young boy is the Guided Body Visit. For this meditation, it's best to lie flat on your back in the "savasana" pose described above. Once you feel your mind has emptied, begin to transport yourself in your mind to a place that makes you feel completely relaxed and content and in harmony, such as lying on a beautiful beach, on the top of a mountain peak, in the woods in a clearing with treetops overhead, or in a green pasture. Create a picture of you being a part of this ideal, peaceful serene environment where you are completely relaxed and content. With each breath, allow your body to feel and hear the same sensations as you would if you were actually in that place.

Using the beach as an example, imagine lying on a soft towel on the warm beach, under an umbrella on a beautiful bright, blue sky. Feel the warmth of the sand underneath you and the sun shining all around you. Feel the cool, refreshing spritzing salty breeze of the ocean mist as it floats into the air and gently covers your body. Hear the gentle rumble of the ocean waves splashing onto the shore, one after another.

Breathe in the air and take in the colors of the scene. (For example, if you are in the mountains, woods, or are in a green grass pasture, breathe in the fresh, crisp air and feel it enter your lungs. Look with amazement at all of the vibrant colors and living species that nature has to offer and observe the unique and special sounds of the birds, insects, and other animals as they speak to each other and to you.)

With each gentle breaking of the waves, your breathing becomes deeper, more relaxed, and your mind brings your body closer to actually being a part of the beach. Begin to snuggle your toes and then your feet beneath the warm, soft beach sand. In the near distance, feel a sense of complete harmony as the waves softly roll onto shore and then retreat back out into the ocean, and just beyond that, you hear the innocent laughter of young children experiencing joy, or the wonderful sounds of the birds singing in harmony with the wind.

Bring in the place that gives you total and complete peace and harmony.

The best part of this meditation is that it can be performed at any time of day, wherever you can find a quiet place to lie down for five-to-fifteen minutes. I enjoy practicing it upon waking in the morning to start my day in harmony, or following my stretching-exercise routine, or to unwind at the end of a busy/hectic day. When I want to positively influence my physical performance—whether at work, before an important presentation, or at an athletic competition—I will perform the Body Visit along with the Mindfulness Awareness Meditation.

MINDFULNESS AWARENESS MEDITATION

This is, by far, my favorite type of emotional/spiritual nourishment when I'm preparing for a performance of any kind. Once I've completed the basic Body Visit or the Guided Body Visit with imagery, as I lie on my back completely relaxed, I place myself in the same naturalistic environment each time to build consistency, which strengthens the effectiveness of the meditation for me. I create an image of me walking in a beautiful, soft, green grass field on a warm sparkling sunny day with weeping willow trees providing occasional overhead shade. I remain captivated by the majestic beauty and the vibrant colors of the rich, dark green grass, the deep blue sky, bright yellow-orange sun, and the exuberant multicolored flowers that are strewn across the pasture.

There is a gentle breeze blowing to keep me cool as I slowly stroll down the green pastures. I am dressed in a loose-fitting soft cotton button-down short-sleeved shirt and comfortably fitted soft cotton shorts. On my feet are open sandals that allow my feet to feel the open air and the warm sun and the soft touch of the grass beneath them.

As I slowly walk down the slopes of the grassy field, I come to a circular cement patio with a beautiful water fountain in the middle. The fountain is surrounded by a waist-high brick foundation with a marble-top finish. As I approach the fountain, I take in the majestic beauty and notice the reflection of the sun sparkling off each water droplet emanating from the fountain as it spouts water out the top. When I reach the fountain, I place my left hand on the cool marble finish atop the brick wall surrounding the fountain and slowly circle the fountain starting on the right side, then I turn back and place my right hand on the marble finish and walk halfway back.

I then continue walking down the grassy green pasture enjoying the cornucopia of colors and fresh smells of the grass, trees, and flowers, and the warmth of the sun on my body. I arrive at another fountain of similar design as the one before. I follow the same movement pattern of walking completely around once from the right side then turning slowly and walking back halfway around in the opposite direction, again placing my right hand atop the marble surface.

I continue with this same pattern of walking down this gently sloping soft bright-green grassy field, passing under the weeping willows that allow the warm sun to peek through the branches while my feet enjoy the softness of the cushioned grass beneath me and the sweet smell of flowers and grass along the way.

The number of fountains that I come across is entirely dependent upon the depth of the meditative state I am seeking to obtain. Regardless of how long I stroll in the grassy field and the number of fountains I come across, my main focus is on the moment and the sensations I experience along the way. In fact, the longer my stroll and time in this meditative state the more I become attuned to other sounds, sights, smells, and happenings around me in nature, such that my awareness becomes super heightened. I begin to notice birds chirping in the trees, the unique colors on the butterflies' wings floating in front of me, and the bees pollinating the flowers along my walk.

Each step brings a greater awareness of my surroundings and things I might not pay attention to any other time in my waking life. It is both exhilarating and entirely relaxing to soak up all the beauty of nature while allowing my body to reach a new state of awareness, focus, and relaxation.

This heightened sense of being is an ideal place to allow the final step of meditation to occur. As I pass by the last fountain in the pasture, I allow myself to enter an environment in which I start off as a spectator in the audience watching a person perform a perfectly executed performance, whatever it might be.

As I'm sitting, observing the performance, without passing any judgment, criticism, or comment, I soon become aware that the person I am observing is me. I sit calmly observing myself perform in an admiring way, passing no judgment, good or bad. I am simply content watching myself perform. The primary reason I sit in content admiration is that my performance is flawless, near-perfect in every way. It does not matter if I am in front of 100,000 people in a packed stadium giving a speech, or performing in an athletic contest.

I am performing effortlessly and am completely calm and content; there is no tension in my body or mind anywhere. I am poised, engaging, and in control no matter the circumstance. If I know who my audience or opponent will be, I anticipate this and put them in the appropriate place and even have them challenge me in some way. My response is always precise, correct, and performed with quiet confidence and poise.

I observe myself from the position of the spectator or audience for the first couple of minutes but then zoom in close to myself and transition into the view of actually performing the action. Similar to my audience view, I perform now as myself and continue to execute and perform with complete effortlessness flow, and with ease and poise.

My breathing, heart rate, and mind are in harmony and rhythmical despite the gravity of the environment that I am performing. I am completely in harmony with the mind, body, and spirit yet fully aware and present at the moment. I call it mind-body-spirit-fullness, and I feel fully integrated as a human being. It's a supreme state of being, one I want to inhabit as often as possible, and I want you to experience this too!

The good news for all of you is, with practice, you can achieve this state in as little as five-to-ten minutes a day.

CULTIVATING A FEELING OF PEACE

Peace comes from cultivating the time to find it. It is there waiting for you at all times if you stop long enough to recognize it. If you don't, then you spin yourself into situations and lives that you would really rather not manifest.

The human body needs its refreshing and restorative sleep, and the proper emotional nurturance as well. If you can incorporate meditations, what you will find is that you will become so much more efficient, focused, and clear. The newly found energy and intent behind your thoughts and actions will help you release anxiety and negative thinking and reach your goals. These are the "golden chains" that Thomas Dekker says keep your body and mind strong, healthy, and connected.

CHAPTER 14

THE PRISE® LIFE IN YOUR POCKET

The future depends on what you do today.
— *Mahatma Gandhi*

What an honor it is to finally share the gifts that have been given to me, the ones that for a long time, even I could not see. What a wild ride these five-and-a-half decades have been, but now I know that as an "archer" my job is to train you to keep your eyes on the PRISE. I believe the evolution of nutrition and applied physiology has just begun!

This book started as a work in progress when I was a young boy searching for meaning and a path in life. Several challenging and early life-transforming events caused me to question my self-worth and identity, but nurturing grandparents, parents, and siblings supported me with their unconditional love and belief in me. My life experiences are the essence of who I am today. During my earlier years, I witnessed some of these same loved ones become ill or diseased. This deeply touched my soul and quickly stoked the flame of my passion and eventual mission in life—to help others live a life of optimal health and peak performance.

For the past thirty years in scientific research, and for almost fifty years of personal experience in nutrition, health, and fitness, this book has taken form. I began my career as a nutrition and applied physiology college professor and scientist, as well as a performance coach, mentor, scientific advisory board member, and leading worldwide expert and spokesperson on nutrition, fitness, and health. These roles have provided me an incredible platform to spread my message, and I am grateful and humbled by each opportunity I'm provided.

Because of a twelve-year insane schedule, I was forced to find a program that would work for all people, at all fitness and weight levels, lacking time in their day. Now, my discoveries can change the world! I can't wait to get out and help others, like you, who are the overstressed working moms; the fathers with too many jobs; the families caring for sick loved ones while trying to stay healthy themselves; the students and athletes driven to be the best while holding down other jobs, and so on.

I have always placed my relationship with others as the most meaningful and fulfilling blessing of what I do. For me, developing a nurturing and caring environment from which to conduct my research, teach my students, coach my athletes, mentor and guide my clients, work alongside colleagues, and motivate my audiences has been at the core of everything I do. It is this atmosphere that has created a rock-solid foundation for The PRISE Life and Protein Pacing Protocol that has served millions and will hopefully serve millions more well into the future.

In the end, as I look back at the incredible nurturing I received from those who saw something in me—something that the world needed—I see how they helped to shape me and therefore shaped this book. Whether it was taking me to play in the garden, or encouraging me to get up in unforgiving weather to go play hockey, or telling me how special I was, when I couldn't see it myself, these things helped me to become the researcher, coach, teacher, and man that I am today. This is powerful. This is humbling, and shows me how important support and encouragement are for each of us.

As I look back on the bad times where I felt humiliated, uninspired, and like I might have blown it, I had the courage to stand back up. This is what I want to give to you. I want you to live a life of optimal health and peak performance. I want you to succeed, and I don't want you to be misled by programs that have no research or proof to back them up.

One of the most valuable psychological lessons we can learn along the way in this life is that we all have deficits. We have strengths, too, but it is amazing to realize that overcoming our deficits is usually what makes us stronger, and is what keeps our hearts pure enough to want to help others. I believe that compassion and humility are the greatest gifts of our Creator.

You may not have had a support system or the love that you needed in the past, but we are a team now, a family. I want you to come read, come play, come learn, come heal, and come achieve. You are safe here. I am here to tell you in no uncertain terms that you are good enough. There is a special path for you, one that brings you health and energy and the life of your dreams.

I hope that after reading this book you are beginning to understand the reason why I thrive on scientific research and why I am so very excited to share my discoveries with the world! I hope I have earned your trust and proven to you that the environment from which I conduct my research, teach my students, coach my athletes, and mentor and guide my clients has been at the core of everything I do. It is this atmosphere that has created a rock-solid foundation for Protein Pacing and The PRISE Life strategies (and PRISE app). I am the actual scientist (with the help of incredible colleagues and research subjects) who made these discoveries and conducted the research that has now been reviewed worldwide. I am cited as the leading authority on nutrition and applied physiology, and I am humbled and honored to be that Dr. Paul.

You now understand how metabolism works, what diet theories are true and which are not, the proper way to exercise without overexertion, how Mother Nature guides us, and how our bodies should really operate. I want you to be truly nourished, emotionally as well as physically, by understanding the value of good nutrition and proper nourishment. No more calorie counting and consuming fake processed food.

Self-care is the new health care, and you must be proactive. By following The PRISE Life, you may live a longer and healthier life. I've tested The PRISE Life Protocol on super-fit men and women, and they outperform their non-PRISE counterparts in every measure of physical performance! This is a lifestyle plan that will work the rest of your life. You can end the diet roller coaster and for the rest of your life follow an excellent, not-too-intense, great-tasting, satiating, never-hungry, "non-diet" eating-for life-program—one that keeps you healthy and does not deprive you.

We, as a society, have to end this deadly cycle of obesity, the rat race of overstress and immobility, the addiction to alcohol and drugs—prescribed or not— which would diminish if we just felt better and could finally claim the ultimate health and peak performance we all so deserve. There is nothing as important as you, your health, and staying motivated so you can achieve all the things you have set out in this lifetime. We deserve to remain as healthy as possible well into our eighties, nineties, and above. Maybe we will become the civilization that heeded the truth and lives to the 120 years we were supposed to live to.

Whether you are running a marathon, are an Olympic athlete, or are just a person hoping to feel their best every day, there is nothing stopping you from not only "keeping your eyes on the prize," but getting and staying there. The power of intention is with you. That intention can become a movement, just as people in the past have been moved when some have been mistreated because of a lack of knowledge. Together, we can be the change agents!

Remember, eat slow, whole and dirty! Nature has been a huge source of inspiration for me. It refreshes me daily with new lessons and provides me with the drive to motivate and help you succeed. Cheers to nature for knowing what we need more than we know ourselves.

The mind, body, and spirit are one, and with the information and discoveries I have been blessed to stumble upon in my research, we can all go out and live balanced, nutritionally supportive lifestyles, which will lead us into the longevity of optimal health and peak performance.

I can't tell you how much I have learned while writing this book. It has been a journey, but I can say that I have evolved because of it. I had my virtue revealed to me during a quantum emergence class and discovered it was "kindness." Which is known as the "attraction" virtue that is based on appreciating and accepting everyone and everything for its existence as equals. My main goal in life is to bring people together and promote equality and fellowship. I've learned even more about myself, and my motivation to share The PRISE Life with everyone in the world is through the roof!

WHERE CAN YOU FIND OUT MORE?

I want you to take a moment, take that champion in you, and go to the computer or grab your smartphone and check out my site: www.priselife.com.

It has all the added pieces that I could not include in this book. Things like: more about The PRISE Life app, lists of all the extensive media coverage of my research (magazines, newspaper, television, radio appearances), and all the peer-reviewed published manuscripts (for all of you analytical folks). These sites include the latest material and updates.

Look through the presentations I have done and find the ones of me on YouTube. Schedule me to come speak to your group. Check out where I will be speaking next and bring your book so I can sign it for you. See my other books: The PRISE Life Handbook, The PRISE Life Playbook, The PRISE Life Cookbook, and The PRISE Life Trainer's Manual.

Although our journey may be coming to an end in this book, I have provided you a roadmap, books, a website, and even an app so that I am always with you. How wonderful is this interlinked world? It is only with your help that I can really achieve my goals over the coming years, to continue investigating lifestyle-related strategies of nutrition, fitness, and mind/body techniques to:

1) Facilitate physical, cognitive, emotional health, and well-being.
2) Prevent cardiovascular, metabolic, cognitive, disease/risk.
3) Optimize physical and athletic performance in people of all ages and health status.

I will devote the rest of my life to being your global content expert and spokesperson for optimizing health and performance through lifestyle strategies of nutrition, fitness, and mind/body techniques.

In my deepest gratitude, I am so happy to welcome you not only to the team, but to your new "PRISE Life," Dr. Paul's family. I know how supportive my current followers are, so I can't wait to have you behind this movement as well. Thank you from the depths of my soul for taking this journey with me. I hope to see you along future paths as they evolve. Know that I am here to serve in whatever capacity can help the most people.

And finally, in closing, as the archer would tell his apprentice, you have been well-trained, grasshopper. Now it is time to go and hit your mark! Keep your eyes on the PRISE! And with the universal ripple effect of the heart that works in gratitude, the mind in clarity, and the spirit in truth, we can change the world.

ACKNOWLEDGMENTS

I am eternally grateful for the love and support of my family and friends, who have always believed in me, in my passions, and in my dedication to helping others live a life of optimal health and peak performance. These are the people who have helped make me the son, brother, teacher, researcher, speaker, husband, father, and man that I am today.

To my mother, Jane Barbara (Petrillo) Arciero, "The eighty-five-year-old hiking grandma," and my father, Donald Vincent Arciero, "Big D," your vibrance, nurturing and love continue to inspire me and create my essence of being. You have my eternal devotion and gratitude.

To my grandfather, John Petrillo, and grandmother, Edith (Deedie) Dean Arciero, whose constant love and belief in me was the turning point of my life on this journey.

To my older brother John, your unwavering love, support, confidence, and mentoring in everything I have done in life has clarified my message for optimal health and peak performance as the world-leading voice.

To my amazing sisters Donna and Jackie, and brothers Chris, Peter, and Matt, combined you created the most wonderful gift of family, love, and support.

To my best friend and beautiful wife, Karen. You've always stood by my side with love, encouragement, and support. You remain the greatest source of my essence, mission (passion), message, and blessing.

To my three amazing and gifted sons Nicholas, Noah, and Aidan. You are the life source of my mission, energy, and motivation and surpass me in every way of existence, matched only by the love we have for each other.

I owe much of my inspiration to carry The PRISE Life message worldwide to the thousands of students in my classes and labs, the athletes I've coached, the hundreds of research study participants, brilliant colleagues, and the millions of people my research, teaching, mentoring, and coaching has influenced over the years.

A special thanks to my good friend Stephen M.R. Covey, whose personal endorsement means everything to me.

A heartfelt thanks to my world-class publishing team at O'Leary Publishing, including one of the most gifted and talented people I know, April O'Leary, and her amazing team member, Heather Davis Desrocher, for the constant support, devotion, and brilliance that they poured into this book. I am grateful for their faith and belief in me as an evangelist and change agent for optimal health and peak performance.

These incredible people have been the driving force behind The PRISE Life and Protein Pacing Protocol. I have been truly blessed with a remarkable team of supporters. I love each one of you with all my heart, mind, and soul.

BIBLIOGRAPHY

2017. http://www.askdrsears.com/topics/feeding-eating/ family-nutrition/ standard-american-diet-sad

2017. https://bionutrient.org/sites/all/files/docs/2011_ Nutrient_Guide.pdf

2017. http://www.wellnessresources.com/weight/articles/ why-toxins-and-waste-products- impede-weight-loss-theleptin-diet-weight "II. Dynamics of Fat Metabolism." How Fat Works. doi:10.4159/9780674045323-004.

"AAAS—The World's Largest General Scientific Society |." AAAS—The World's Largest General Scientific Society |. March 15, 1970. Accessed February 17, 2018. https://www. aaas.org/https://www.aaas.org/sites/default/files/Agencies.

"A better way to exercise." Skidmore College. Accessed November 24, 2017. http:// www. skidmore.edu/news/2014/092314-a-better-way-to-exercise.php.

"ACSM | History." American College of Sports Medicine. Accessed February 23, 2018. http:// www.acsm.org/about-acsm/who-we-are/history.

"ACSM | OMHA Reference Search—Chronological Search by Author." American College of Sports Medicine. Accessed February 23, 2018. http://www. acsm. org/public-information/health-physical-activity-reference-database/ omha-reference-search---chronological-search-by-author.

"A Sleepless Night Can Wreck Your DNA." Daily Mail (London), July 23, 2015.

Allport, Susan. The Queen of Fats: Why Omega-3s Were Removed from the Western Diet and What We Can Do to Replace Them. Berkeley, CA: University of California Press, 2006.

"Abraham-Hicks Publications." Home of Abraham-Hicks Law of Attraction—It All Started Here! Accessed January 14, 2018. http://www.abraham-hicks.com/ lawofattractionsource/index.php?i=4.

"Abraham-Hicks Sessions." Abraham-Hicks Sessions. Accessed February 1, 2018. https://abrahamhickssessions.wordpress.com//2014/07/11/ metabolism-is-vibrational-response-2/.

Anderson, E. N. Everyone Eats: Understanding Food and Culture. 2nd ed. New York: New York University Press, 2014. Anderson-Hanley, Cay, and Paul Arciero. "Seniors Cybercycling for Enhanced Cognitive Performance." PsycEXTRA Dataset. doi:10.1037/ e530522011-009.

Anderson-Hanley C., Paul J. Arciero, Nicole Barcelos, Joseph Nimon, Tracey Rocha, Marisa Thurin and Molly Maloney. "Executive function and self-regulated exergaming adherence among older adults." Frontiers in Human Neuroscience. Dec. 2014; Volume 8, Article 989.

Anderson-Hanley, C., P. J. Arciero, A. M. Brickman, J. P. Nimon, N. Okuma, S. C. Westen, M.

E. Merz, B. D. Pence, J. A. Woods, A. F. Kramer, and E. A. Zimmerman. "Exergaming and older adult cognition: a cluster-randomized clinical trial." American Journal of Preventive Medicine. February 2012. Accessed March 20, 2018. https://www.ncbi.nlm.nih.gov/ pubmed/22261206.

Anshel, Mark H. Applied Exercise Psychology: A Practitioner's Guide to Improving Client Health and Fitness. New York: Springer Publishing Company, 2006.

Aragon, Alan A. Brad J. Schoenfeld, Robert Wildman, Susan Kleiner, Trisha VanDusseldorp, Lem Taylor, Conrad P. Earnest, Paul J. Arciero, Colin Wilborn, Douglas S. Kalman, Jeffrey

R. Stout, Darryn S. Willoughby, Bill Campbell, Shawn M. Arent, Laurent Bannock, Abbie E. Smith-Ryan and Jose Antonio. "International society of sports nutrition position stand: Diets and Body Composition." J Int Soc Sports Nutr. 201714:16. DOI: 10.1186/ s12970-017-0174-y.

"Arciero P - PubMed - NCBI." National Center for Biotechnology Information. Accessed March 16, 2018. https://www.ncbi.nlm.nih.gov/pubmed/?term=arciero%2Bp.

Arciero, Paul. "GenioFit on the App Store." App Store. July 08, 2016. Accessed January 8, 2018. https://itunes.apple.com/us/app/geniofit/id1087668497?mt=8. The 2018 App is now PRISE Fitness App (www.prisewell.com).

Arciero, PJ, et al. "Effects of caffeine ingestion on NE kinetics, fat oxidation, and energy expenditure in younger and older men." Am. J. Physiol. 268 (Endocrinol. Metab. 31): Ell92- El198 1995.

Arciero PJ, Baur D, Connelly S, Ormsbee MJ. "Timed-daily ingestion of whey protein and exercise training reduces visceral adipose tissue mass and improves insulin resistance: The PRISE Study." J Appl Physiol (1985). 2014 Jul 1;117(1):1-10

Arciero, PJ. Christopher L. Bougopoulos, Bradley C. Nindl, and Neal L. Benowitz. "Influence of Age on the Thermic Response to Caffeine in Women." Metabolism, Vol49, No 1

(January), 2000: pp 101-107.

Arciero PJ, Edmonds RC, Bunsawat K, Gentile CL, Ketcham C, Darin C, Renna M, Zheng Q, Zhang JZ, Ormsbee MJ. "Protein-Pacing from Food or

Supplementation Improves Physical Performance in Overweight Men and Women: The PRISE 2 Study." Nutrients. 2016 May 11;8(5)

Arciero, Paul J., and Michael J. Ormsbee. "Relationship of blood pressure, behavioral mood state, and physical activity following caffeine ingestion in younger and older women." Applied Physiology, Nutrition, and Metabolism 34, no. 4 (2009): 754-62. doi:10.1139/ h09-068.

Arciero, PJ, et al. "Relationship of blood pressure, heart rate and behavioral mood state to norepinephrine kinetics in younger and older men following caffeine ingestion." European Journal of Clinical Nutrition 52, no. 11 (1998): 805-12. doi:10.1038/sj.ejcn.1600651.

Arciero PJ, Gentile CL, Martin-Pressman R, Ormsbee MJ, Everett M, Zwicky L, Steele CA. "Increased dietary protein and combined high intensity aerobic and resistance exercise improve body fat distribution and cardiovascular risk factors." Int J Sport Nutr Exerc Metab. 2006 Aug;16(4):373-92.

Arciero PJ, Gentile CL, Pressman R, Everett M, Ormsbee MJ, Martin J, Santamore J, Gorman L, Fehling PC, Vukovich MD, Nindl BC. "Moderate protein intake improves total and regional body composition and insulin sensitivity in overweight adults." Metabolism. 2008 Jun;57(6):757-65.

Arciero, PJ, et al. "Resting metabolic rate is lower in women than in men." Journal of Applied Physiology 75, no. 6 (1993): 2514-520. doi:10.1152/jappl.1993.75.6.2514.

Arciero PJ, Hannibal NS, Nindl BC, Gentile CL, Hamed J, Vukovich MD. "Comparison of creatine ingestion and resistance training on energy expenditure and limb blood flow." Metabolism: Clinical and Experimental, vol 50: pp 1429-1434, 2001.

Arciero PJ, Ives SJ, Norton C, Escudero D, Minicucci O, O'Brien G, Paul M, Ormsbee MJ, Miller V, Sheridan C, He F. "Protein-Pacing and Multi-Component Exercise Training Improves Physical Performance Outcomes in Exercise-Trained Women: The PRISE 3 Study." Nutrients. 2016 Jun 1;8(6)

Arciero PJ, Miller VJ, Ward E. "Performance Enhancing Diets and the PRISE Protocol to Optimize Athletic Performance." J Nutr Metab. 2015;2015:715859

Arciero PJ, Ormsbee MJ, Gentile CL, Nindl BC, Brestoff JR, Ruby M. "Increased protein intake and meal frequency reduces abdominal fat during energy balance and energy deficit." Obesity (Silver Spring). 2013 Jul;21(7):1357-66

Arciero PJ, Smith DL, Calles-Escandon J. "Effects of inactivity on glucose tolerance, energy expenditure, and blood flow in highly trained endurance athletes." J Appl Physiol, 1998; 84:1217-1224.

Arciero PJ, Vukovich MD, Holloszy JO, Racette S, Kohrt WM. "Comparison of a short- term diet and exercise training on insulin action in individuals with abnormal glucose tolerance." J Appl Physiol. 86(6): 1930-1935, 1999.

Arciero, Paul, Rohan Edmonds, Feng He, Emery Ward, Eric Gumpricht, Alex Mohr, Michael Ormsbee, and Arne Astrup. "Protein-Pacing Caloric-Restriction Enhances Body Composition Similarly in Obese Men and Women during Weight Loss and Sustains Efficacy during Long-Term Weight Maintenance." Nutrients 8, no. 8 (2016): 476. doi:10.3390/nu8080476.

Areta, J.L.; Burke, L.M.; Camera, D.M.; West, D.W.; Crawshay, S.; Moore, D.R.; Stellingwerff, T.; Phillips, S.M.; Hawley, J.A.; Coffey, V.G. "Reduced resting skeletal muscle protein synthesis is rescued by resistance exercise and protein ingestion following short-term energy deficit." Am. J. Physiol. Endocrinol. Metab. 2014, 306, 989–997.

Astrup, A.; Raben, A.; Geiker, N. "The role of higher protein diets in weight control and obesity-related comorbidities." Int. J. Obes. 2014, 39, 721–726.

Bajarin, Tim. "Fitbit: Here's Why Fitness Trackers Are Here to Stay." Time. June 24, 2015. Accessed March 3, 2018. http://time.com/3934258/ fitness-trackers-fitbit/?xid=emailshare.

Barcelos, Nicole, Nikita Shah, Katherine Cohen, Michael J. Hogan, Eamon Mulkerrin, Paul

J. Arciero, Brian D. Cohen, Arthur F. Kramer, and Cay Anderson-Hanley. "Aerobic and Cognitive Exercise (ACE) Pilot Study for Older Adults: Executive Function Improves with Cognitive Challenge While Exergaming." JINS, 21: 10; 768-779, 2015.

Barrett, Julia R. "The Science of Soy: What Do We Really Know?" Environmental Health Perspectives 114, no. 6 (2006): A352+.

Batacan, Romeo B., Mitch J. Duncan, Vincent J. Dalbo, Patrick S. Tucker, and Andrew S. Fenning. "Effects of high-intensity interval training on cardiometabolic health: a systematic review and meta-analysis of intervention studies." British Journal of Sports Medicine 51, no. 6 (2016): 494-503. doi:10.1136/bjsports-2015-095841.

Baum, J. I., M. Gray, and A. Binns. "Breakfasts Higher in Protein Increase Postprandial Energy Expenditure, Increase Fat Oxidation, and Reduce Hunger in Overweight Children from 8 to 12 Years of Age." The Journal of Nutrition. October 2015. Accessed January 22, 2018. https://www.ncbi.nlm.nih.gov/ pubmed/26269241.

Berardi, Ph.D. John. "Breakfast: Not Really the Most Important Meal of the Day." The Huffington Post. December 15, 2013. Accessed March 18, 2018. https://www. huffingtonpost.com/john-berardi-phd/breakfast-health_b_4436439.html.

Berger, Vance W., and A. J. Sankoh. "Prognostic Variables in Clinical Trials." Methods and Applications of Statistics in Clinical Trials, 2014, 789-98. doi:10.1002/9781118596005.ch67.

Bergman, Bryan C., Leigh Perreault, Allison Strauss, Samantha Bacon, Anna Kerege, Kathleen Harrison, Joseph T. Brozinick, Devon M. Hunerdosse, Mary C.

Playdon, William Holmes, Hai Hoang Bui, Phil Sanders, Parker Siddall, Tao Wei, Melissa K. Thomas, Ming Shang Kuo, and Robert H. Eckel. "Intramuscular triglyceride synthesis: the importance of muscle lipid partitioning in humans." American Journal of Physiology-Endocrinology and Metabolism 314, no. 2 (2018). doi:10.1152/ajpendo.00142.2017.

"Best Way to Slow Aging? High-Intensity Interval Training Exercise—but Not Just Any Kind."

The Buffalo News (Buffalo, NY), April 15, 2017.

"Biochemistry & Molecular Biology." Michigan Academician 37, no. 4 (2008): 10+. Boecker, H., T. Sprenger, M. E. Spilker, G. Henriksen, M. Koppenhoefer, K. J. Wagner, M.

Valet, A. Berthele, and T. R. Tolle. "The runner's high: opioidergic mechanisms in the human brain." Cerebral Cortex (New York, NY:1991). November 2008. Accessed March 20, 2018. https://www.ncbi.nlm.nih.gov/pubmed/18296435.

Bugaut, M. "Occurrence, Absorption, and Metabolism of Short Chain Fatty Acids in the Digestive Tract of Mammals." Comparative Biochemistry and Physiology. B,

Comparative Biochemistry. Accessed March 5, 2018. https://www.ncbi.nlm.nih.gov/pubmed/3297476.

Burke, Louise, and Greg Cox. The Complete Guide to Food for Sports Performance: A Guide to Peak Nutrition for Your Sport. 3rd ed. Crow's Nest, N.S.W.: Allen & Unwin, 2010.

"CDC Newsroom." Centers for Disease Control and Prevention. July 18, 2017. Accessed February 23, 2018. https://www.cdc.gov/media/releases/2017/p0718-diabetes-report. html.

"Carbohydrates and Resistant Starch May Help Weight Loss." Time. Accessed November 22, 2017. http://time.com/4318201/carbohydrates-weight-loss-resistant-starch/.

Case, Meredith A. "Accuracy of Devices to Track Physical Activity Data." JAMA. February 10, 2015. Accessed March 3, 2018. https://jamanetwork.com/journals/jama/ fullarticle/2108876#tab1.

Centers for Disease Control and Prevention. June 02, 2009. Accessed February 18, 2018. https://www.cdc.gov/nchs/data/hus/hus16.pdf#056.

Chaput, J-P Després, C. Bouchard, and A. Tremblay. "Longer sleep duration associates with lower adiposity gain in adult short sleepers." Nature News. June 07, 2011. Accessed March 1, 2018. http://www.nature.com/articles/ijo2011110.

Chaput, Jean-Philippe, Jessica McNeil, Jean-Pierre Després, Claude Bouchard, and Angelo Tremblay. "Seven to Eight Hours of Sleep a Night Is Associated with a Lower Prevalence of the Metabolic Syndrome and Reduced Overall

Cardiometabolic Risk in Adults." PLOS ONE. Accessed March 11, 2018. http://journals.plos.org/plosone/ article?id=10.1371%2Fjournal.pone.0072832.

Cheeke, P. R., and E. S. Dierenfeld. "Fat and fatty acid metabolism." Comparative animal nutrition and metabolism: 133-44. doi:10.1079/9781845936310.0133.

Cheikh Rouhou, M.; Karelis, A.D.; St-Pierre, D.H.; Lamontagne, L. "Adverse effects of weight loss: Are persistent organic pollutants a potential culprit?" Diabetes Metab. 2016, 42, 215–223.

Chivian, Eric, Aaron Bernstein, and Kofi Annan, eds. Sustaining Life: How Human Health Depends on Biodiversity. New York: Oxford University Press, 2008.

"Clean Your Body's Drains: 10 Ways to Detoxify Your Lymphatic System." 2017.

Healthy and Natural World. http://www.healthyandnaturalworld.com/ natural-ways-to-cleanse-your-lymphatic-system/

Clifton, P.M.; Bastiaans, K.; Keogh, J.B. "High protein diets decrease total and abdominal fat and improve CVD risk profile in overweight and obese men and women with elevated triacylglycerol." Nutr. Metab. Cardiovasc. Dis. 2009, 19, 548–554.

Connor, Erinn. "Be Aware of the Sleep-Weight Connections." The Record (Bergen County, NJ), March 7, 2013.

Cotterill, Stewart. Team Psychology in Sports: Theory and Practice. New York: Routledge, 2012. Cui, Yufei, Kaijun Niu, Cong Huang, Haruki Momma, Lei Guan, Hui Guo, Masahiko Chujo,

Atsushi Otomo, and Ryoichi Nagatomi. "Relationship between daily isoflavone intake and sleep in Japanese adults: a cross-sectional study." Nutrition Journal. December 29, 2015. Accessed March 3, 2018. https://nutritionj.biomedcentral.com/articles/10.1186/ s12937-015-0117-x.

"Dairy Processing Handbook." Dairy Processing Handbook. Accessed February 11, 2018. http://dairyprocessinghandbook.com/chapter/whey-processing.

Diamond, Dan. "Just 8% of People Achieve Their New Year's Resolutions. Here's How They Do It." Forbes. January 02, 2013. Accessed January 14, 2018. https://www.forbes.com/sites/dandiamond/2013/01/01/

just-8-of-people-achieve-their-new-years-resolutions-heres-how-they-did-it/2/. "Dimethyl Sulfoxide (DMSO) and Methylsulfonylmethane (MSM) for Osteoarthritis."

National Center for Complementary and Integrative Health. September 24, 2017. Accessed February 23, 2018. https://nccih.nih.gov/health/supplements/dmso-msm.

Dansinger, M.L.; Gleason, J.A.; Griffith, J.L.; Selker, H.P.; Schaefer, E.J. "Comparison of the Atkins, Ornish, Weight Watchers, and Zone diets for weight loss and heart disease risk reduction: A randomized trial." J. Am. Med. Assoc. 2005, 293, 43–53.

"Definition." American Society of Exercise Physiologists. Accessed December 18, 2017. https://www.asep.org/about-asep/definition/.

"Digesting 'Fat Chance' and Understanding Obesity." Daily Herald (Arlington Heights, IL), January 30, 2013.

"Digital Object Identifier System." Digital Object Identifier System. Accessed December 19, 2017. https://doi.org/10.1080/00336297.2007.10483534.

"Dr. Arciero: Losing Weight & Keeping it Off - Isagenix Podcast." The Official Isagenix Podcast Site. August 11, 2017. Accessed November 24, 2017. http://isagenixpodcast. com/dr-arciero-losing-weight-keeping-off/.

"Dr. Paul Arciero, Skidmore College." WAMC. Accessed November 28, 2017. http://wamc. org/post/dr-paul-arciero-skidmore-college.

DrPaulsProtocol. "Dr. Paul Arciero." YouTube. Accessed November 25, 2017. http://www. youtube.com/user/DrPaulsProtocol.

Dirinck, E.L.; Dirtu, A.C.; Govindan, M.; Covaci, A.; Jorens, P.G.; van Gaal, L.F. "Endocrine-disrupting polychlorinated biphenyls in metabolically healthy and unhealthy obese subjects before and after weight loss: Difference at the start but not at the finish." Am. J. Clin. Nutr. 2016, 103, 989–998.

Dirinck, E.; Dirtu, A.C.; Jorens, P.G.; Malarvannan, G.; Covaci, A.; Van Gaal, L.F. "Pivotal role for the visceral fat compartment in the release of persistent organic pollutants during weight loss." J. Clin. Endocrinol. Metab. 2015, 100, 4463–4471.

DrugWatch. July 29, 2015. Accessed January 8, 2018. https://www.drugwatch. com/2015/07/29/drug-abuse-in-america/.

"Eating More Can Help You to Lose Weight. Understand Your Body and Change Your Life."

Daily Mail (London), April 14, 1997.

"Eight Eating Habits You Need to Break." The Buffalo News (Buffalo, NY), August 22, 2015. Elder, Charles R., Christina M. Gullion, Kristine L. Funk, Lynn L. DeBar, Nangel M.

Lindberg, and Victor J. Stevens. International Journal of Obesity (2005). January 2012. Accessed March 20, 2018. https://www.ncbi.nlm.nih.gov/pmc/articles/PMC3136584/.

Elkins, Chris. "Hooked on Pharmaceuticals: Prescription Drug Abuse in America."

Evans, Malkanthi, John Rumberger, Isao Azumano, Joseph Napolitano, Danielle Citrolo, and Toshikazu Kamiya. "Pantethine, a derivative of vitamin B5, favorably alters total, LDL and non-HDL cholesterol in low to moderate cardiovascular risk subjects eligible for statin therapy: a triple-blinded placebo and diet-controlled investigation." Vascular Health and Risk Management, 2014, 89. doi:10.2147/vhrm.s57116.

"EXERCISE PHYSIOLOGY." Ece Soccer. Accessed December 15, 2017. http://ece-soccer.com/dt_activities/physiology/.

"Exergaming and Older Adult Cognition: A Cluster Randomized Clinical Trial." American Journal of Preventive Medicine. January 16, 2012. Accessed March 20, 2018. https://www. sciencedirect.com/science/article/pii/S0749379711008622.

Farahbakhsh-Farsi, Payam, Abolghassem Djazayery, Mohammad Reza Eshraghian,

Fariba Koohdani, Mahnaz Zarei, Mohammad Hassan Javanbakht, Hoda Derakhshanian, and Mahmoud Djalali. "Effect of Omega-3 Supplementation on Lipocalin 2 and Retinol- Binding Protein 4 in Type 2 Diabetic Patients." Iranian Journal of Public Health 45, no. 1 (2016): 63+.

"Fat and Calories." Cleveland Clinic. Accessed January 9, 2018. https://my.clevelandclinic.org/health/articles/4182-fat-and-calories.

"Fat May Spur Heart Cells on to Suicide." Science News, May 12, 2001.

Feudtner, Chris. Bittersweet: Diabetes, Insulin, and the Transformation of Illness. Edited by Allan

M. Brandt and Larry R. Churchill. Chapel Hill, NC: University of North Carolina Press, 2003.

"Fiber and Saturated Fat Are Associated with Sleep Arousals and Slow Wave." National Center for Biotechnology Information. Accessed March 3, 2018. https://www.ncbi.nlm.nih.gov/ pubmed.

Fossel, Michael B. Cells, Aging, and Human Disease. New York: Oxford University Press, 2004. Franz, M.J.; Van Wormer, J.J.; Crain, A.L.; Boucher, J.L.; Histon, T.; Caplan, W.; Bowman, J.D.;

Pronk, N.P. "Weight-loss outcomes: A systematic review and meta-analysis of weight-loss clinical trials with a minimum 1-year follow-up." J. Am. Diet. Assoc. 2007, 107, 1755–1767.

Gaidos, Susan. "Fat as a Fixer: Adipose Tissue Is a Natural Storehouse of Healing Cells."

Science News, March 19, 2016, 22+.

Gardner, C.D.; Kiazand, A.; Alhassan, S.; Kim, S.; Stafford, R.S.; Balise, R.R.; Kraemer, H.C.; King, A.C. "Comparison of the Atkins, Zone, Ornish, and LEARN diets for change in weight and related risk factors among overweight premenopausal women: The A TO Z Weight Loss Study: A randomized trial." J. Am. Med. Assoc. 2007, 297, 969–977.

Gardner, C. D., J. F. Trepanowski, L. C. Del, M. E. Hauser, J. Rigdon, J. P. Ioannidis, M. Desai, and A. C. King. "Effect of Low-Fat vs Low-Carbohydrate Diet on 12-Month Weight Loss in Overweight Adults and the Association With

Genotype Pattern or Insulin Secretion: The DIETFITS Randomized Clinical Trial." JAMA. February 20, 2018. Accessed March 26, 2018. https://www.ncbi. nlm.nih.gov/pubmed/29466592.

"GenioFit—The guide to getting you there." GenioFit. Accessed November 24, 2017. http:// www.geniofit.com/. The 2018 App is now PRISE Fitness App (www. prisewell.com).

Genné-Bacon, Elizabeth A. The Yale Journal of Biology and Medicine. June 2014. Accessed January 18, 2018. https://www.ncbi.nlm.nih.gov/pmc/articles/ PMC4031802/.

Gentile, Christopher L., Emery Ward, Jens Juul Holst, Arne Astrup, Michael J. Ormsbee, Scott Connelly, and Paul J. Arciero. "Resistant starch and protein intake enhance fat oxidation and feelings of fullness in lean and overweight/ obese women." Nutrition Journal.

October 29, 2015. Accessed January 20, 2018. https://nutritionj.biomedcentral.com/ articles/10.1186/s12937-015-0104-2.

Gibbons, Ann, and Matthieu Paley. "The Evolution of Diet." National Geographic.

Accessed January 18, 2018. https://www.nationalgeographic.com/foodfeatures/ evolution-of-diet/.

Gluckman, Peter, and Mark Hanson. Mismatch: Why Our World No Longer Fits Our Bodies.

New York: Oxford University Press, 2006.

Goho, Alexandra. "Our Microbes, Ourselves: How Bacterial Communities in the Body Influence Human Health." Science News, May 19, 2007, 314+.

"GoodTherapy.org." Erik Erikson Biography. Accessed January 8, 2018. https://www. goodtherapy.org/famous-psychologists/erik-erikson.html.

Google. Accessed March 17, 2018. https://scholar.google.com/ scholar?start=0&q=arciero pj&hl=en&as_sdt=0,3.

Grey, Jennie. "Students in Saratoga Springs High School's new nutrition class tour Skidmore College labs." The Saratogian. October 22, 2012. Accessed March 10, 2018. http://www. saratogian.com/article/ST/20121022/NEWS/310229936.

"Guide to Healthy Drinks." www.be-fit.me. Accessed March 10, 2018. http://www. be-fit.me/ guide-to-healthy-drinks-411/.

Harris, Herbert W., Pranay Jaiswal, Valerie Holmes, Richard H. Weisler, and Ashwin A. Patkar. "Vitamin D Deficiency and Psychiatric Illness: Supplementation Might

Help Patients with Depression, Seasonal Mood Disturbances." Current Psychiatry 12, no. 4 (2013): 18+.

He, Feng, Li Zuo, Emery Ward, and Paul Arciero. "Serum Polychlorinated Biphenyls Increase and Oxidative Stress Decrease with a Protein-Pacing

Caloric Restriction Diet in Obese Men and Women." International Journal of Environmental Research and Public Health 14, no. 12 (2017): 59. doi:10.3390/ijerph14010059.

Health A-Z. Accessed January 9, 2018. http://www.betterlifeunlimited.com/healthnews/health_az/issues/macronutrients

_carbohydrates_proteins_and_fats.aspx.

Hefferon, Kathleen. Let Thy Food Be Thy Medicine: Plants and Modern Medicine. New York: Oxford University Press, 2012.

Heymsfield, S.B.; Harp, J.B.; Reitman, M.L.; Beetsch, J.W.; Schoeller, D.A.; Erondu, N.; Pietrobelli, A. "Why do obese patients not lose more weight when treated with low- calorie diets? A mechanistic perspective." Am. J. Clin. Nutr. 2007, 85, 346–354.

"History of Psychology (387 BC to Present)." AllPsych. Accessed February 22, 2018. https:// allpsych.com/timeline/.

Hopper, Christopher A., Bruce Fisher, and Kathy D. Munoz. Physical Activity and Nutrition for Health. Champaign, IL: Human Kinetics, 2008.

"How to exercise less and get better results." All 4 Women. June 03, 2014.

Accessed March 10, 2018. https://www.all4women.co.za/211583/health/ how-to-exercise-less-and-get-better-results.

"How to get into the best shape of your life, according to science." Fox News. Accessed March 10, 2018. http://www.foxnews.com/lifestyle/2017/04/06/how-to-get-into-best-shape- your-life-according-to-science.html.

Howell, S., and R. Kones. "Calories In, Calories Out" and Macronutrient Intake: The Hope, Hype, and Science of Calories." American Journal of Physiology, Endocrinology, and Metabolism. November 01, 2017. Accessed March 26, 2018. https://www.ncbi.nlm.nih. gov/pubmed/28765272.

Hunter, Beatrice Trum. "The Form Counts: Proteins, Fats and Carbohydrates."

Consumers' Research Magazine, August 2001.

Imbeault, P.; Tremblay, A.; Simoneau, J.A.; Joanisse, D.R. "Weight loss-induced rise in plasma pollutant is associated with reduced skeletal muscle oxidative capacity." Am. J. Physiol.

Endocrinol. Metab. 2002, 282, E574–E579.

"Inflammation and Its Diseases." Nutrition Health Review, January 1, 2013, 2+. "Is breakfast really the most important meal? Why a new study says maybe not."

TODAY.com. Accessed March 18, 2018. https://www.today.com/health/ new-study-says-breakfast-may-not-be-most-important-meal-t37991.

"Is Soy Bad for You?—Dr. Axe." 2017. Dr. Axe. https:// draxe.com/is-soy-bad-for-you/

Ives SJ, Bloom S, Matias A, Morrow N, Martins N, Roh Y, Ebenstein D, O'Brien G, Escudero D, Brito K, Glickman L, Connelly S, Arciero PJ (Senior Corresponding

Author). "Effects of a combined protein and antioxidant supplement on the recovery of muscle function and soreness following eccentric exercise." J Int Soc Sports Nutr. 2017 July 3;14:21.

Ives SJ, Norton C, Miller V, Minicucci O, Robinson J, O'Brien G, Escudero D, Paul M, Sheridan C, Curran K, Rose K, Robinson N, He F, Arciero PJ. "Multi-modal exercise training and protein-pacing enhances physical performance adaptations independent of growth hormone and BDNF but may be dependent on IGF-1 in exercise-trained men." Growth Horm IGF Res. 2017 Feb;32:60-70.

R. Jäger, et al... "International Society of Sports Nutrition Position Stand: Protein and Exercise." J Int Soc Sports Nutr. 201714:20 DOI: 10.1186/s12970-017-0177-8.

Jahnke, Art. "Who Picks Up the Tab for Science?" History and Future of Funding for Scientific   Research | Research. Accessed January 8, 2018. http://www.bu.edu/ research/articles/funding-for-scientific-research/.

Jeffers, Glenn. "Training for a Marathon. (Body Talk: Black Health and Fitness)." Ebony, March 2003, 86+.

Johansen, Bruce E. The Dirty Dozen: Toxic Chemicals and the Earth's Future. Westport, CT: Praeger, 2003.

Kadey, Matthew. "Attack of the Diet Saboteurs." Vegetarian Times, January/February 2015, 70+.

Kelli, Heval Mohamed, Frank Corrigan, Robert Heinl, Devinder Dhindsa, Muhammad Hammadah, Ayman Samman-Tahhan, Pratik Sandesara, Talal Alghamdi, Ibhar Al Mheid, Yi-An Ko, Thomas Ziegler, Laurence Sperling, Kenneth Brigham, Dean Jones, Viola Vaccarino, Greg Martin, and Arshed Quyyumi. "Changes in Body Fat Distribution Is Associated with Oxidative Stress." Journal of the American College of Cardiology 69, no. 11 (2017): 1795. doi:10.1016/s0735-1097(17)35184-7.

Kerksick, Chad; Shawn Arent; Brad J Schoenfeld; Jeffrey R Stout; Bill Campbell; Colin Wilborn; Lem Taylor; Doug Kalman; Abbie E Smith-Ryan; Richard B Kreider; Darryn Willoughby; Paul J. Arciero; Trisha VanDusseldorp; Mike Ormsbee; Robert Wildman; Mike Greenwood; Tim Ziegenfuss; Alan A Aragon; Jose Antonio. "International Society of Sports Nutrition Position Stand: Nutrient Timing." J Int Soc Sports Nutr. 14:33 https:// doi.org/10.1186/s12970-017-0189-4.

Kinsey, A. W., Eddy, W., Madzima, T., Panton, L., Arciero, P.J., Kim, J-S, & Ormsbee, M. J. "The Influence of Nighttime Protein and Carbohydrate Intake on Appetite and Cardiometabolic Risk in Sedentary Overweight and Obese Women." Br J Nutr, 2015. Tyler Graham."Laird Hamilton's Bulletproof Coffee Breakfast Recipe." Men's Journal. December 05, 2017. Accessed March 10, 2018. https://www.mensjournal.com/   health-fitness/bulletproof-coffee-the-new-power-breakfast-20141117/.

Larsen, T.M.; Dalskov, S.; van Baak, M.; Jebb, S.A.; Papadaki, A.; Pfeiffer, A.F.H.; Martinez, J.A.; Handjieva-Darlenska, T.; Kunesova, M.; Pihlsgard, M.; et al. "Diets with high or low protein content and glycemic index for weight-loss maintenance." N. Engl. J. Med. 2010, 363, 2102–2113.

Lawrence, Glen D. The Fats of Life: Essential Fatty Acids in Health and Disease. New Brunswick, NJ: Rutgers University Press, 2010.

"Learn about Dioxin." EPA. March 22, 2017. Accessed February 25, 2018. https://www.epa. gov/dioxin/learn-about-dioxin.

Lees, A., I. Maynard, M. Hughes, and T. Reilly, eds. Science and Racket Sports II. London: E & FN Spon, 1998.

Lees, A., J.-F. Kahn, and I. W. Maynard. Science and Racket Sports III. New York: Routledge, 2004.

Leidy, H. J., H. A. Hoertel, S. M. Douglas, K. A. Higgins, and R. S. Shafer. "A high-protein breakfast prevents body fat gain, through reductions in daily intake and hunger, in 'Breakfast skipping' adolescents." Obesity (Silver Spring, Md.). September 2015. Accessed March 18, 2018. https://www.ncbi.nlm.nih.gov/pubmed/26239831.

Levine, James A. "Non-exercise activity thermogenesis (NEAT)." Best Practice & Research Clinical Endocrinology & Metabolism 16, no. 4 (2002): 679-702. doi:10.1053/ beem.2002.0227.

MacMillan, Amanda. "Why Athletes Should Use Caffeine Patches." Outside Online. April 12, 2017. Accessed March 10, 2018. https://www.outsideonline. com/1786291/

are-caffeine-patches-safe-athletes.

Manninen, Anssi H. Journal of the International Society of Sports Nutrition. 2004. Accessed March 3, 2018. https://www.ncbi.nlm.nih.gov/pmc/articles/PMC2129159/.

Manton, Catherine. Fed Up: Women and Food in America. Westport, CT: Bergin & Garvey, 1999.

Martarelli, Daniele, Mario Cocchioni, Stefania Scuri, and Pierluigi Pompei. Evidence-based Complementary and Alternative Medicine: eCAM. 2011. Accessed March 20, 2018. https://www.ncbi.nlm.nih.gov/pmc/articles/PMC3139518/.

"Medical News Today." Medical News Today. Accessed February 11, 2018. https://www. medicalnewstoday.com/articles/263371.php.

"Meditation-based Program Unveiled for Tennis Players." International Journal of Humanities and Peace 19, no. 1 (2003): 103.

Mednick, Sara C., Nicholas A. Christakis, and James H. Fowler. "The Spread of Sleep Loss Influences Drug Use in Adolescent Social Networks." PLOS ONE. Accessed

March 1, 2018. http://journals.plos.org/plosone/article?id=10.1371%2Fjournal. pone.0009775.

"Miracle tricks to burning calories." IOL Lifestyle. November 13, 2016. Accessed March 10, 2018. https://www.iol.co.za/lifestyle/health/miracle-tricks-to-burning-calories-623661.

Mosher, Rachel, Kyler Crawford, and Andrea Lukowiak. "A Soy-Based Alternative to Traditional Bacterial Nutrient Media." The American Biology Teacher 71, no. 1 (2009): 49+.

Mozaffarian, Dariush. "US Dietary Guidelines and Lifting the Total Dietary Fat Ban." JAMA. June 23, 2015. Accessed February 25, 2018. https://jamanetwork. com/journals/jama/ article-abstract/2338262?resultClick=3&redirect=true.

"National Center for Biotechnology Information." National Center for Biotechnology Information. Accessed February 11, 2018. https://www.ncbi.nlm.nih.gov/pmc/ articles/ PMC3905294/.

"National Center for Health Statistics." Centers for Disease Control and Prevention. March 17, 2017. Accessed February 23, 2018. https://www.cdc.gov/nchs/fastats/ leading-causes-of- death.htm.

Nestle, Marion. Food Politics: How the Food Industry Influences Nutrition and Health. Revised ed. Berkeley, CA: University of California Press, 2013.

"New Isagenix Study Findings on Weight Loss and Toxins." Isagenix Health. March 15, 2017. Accessed November 24, 2017. http://www.isagenixhealth.net/ new-Isagenix-study-findings-weight-loss-toxins/.

OECD. "OECD Statistics." OECD Statistics. Accessed March 7, 2018. https://stats. oecd.org/. "Opioid Overdose." Centers for Disease Control and Prevention. August 30, 2017. Accessed

January 8, 2018. https://www.cdc.gov/drugoverdose/epidemic/index.html.

Ormsbee MJ & Arciero PJ (Senior Corresponding Author). "Detraining Increases Body Fat and Weight and Decreases VO2peak and Metabolic Rate." J Strength Cond Res, 26(8): 2087-2095, 2012.

Ormsbee MJ, Kinsey AW, Eddy WR, Madzima TA, Arciero PJ, Panton LB. "The influence of exercise training and nighttime eating in overweight and obese women." Appl. Physiol. Nutr. Metab. 40: 1–9 (2015)

"Overweight & Obesity." Centers for Disease Control and Prevention. August 31, 2017.

Accessed February 25, 2018. https://www.cdc.gov/obesity/data/prevalence-maps. html. "Paul J Arciero." Paul J Arciero - The Obesity Society. Accessed November 24, 2017. http://

www.obesity.org/content/paul-arciero.

"Paul J Arciero | Publications - ResearchGate." Accessed November 24, 2017. https:// www. bing.com/Paul_Arciero publications,5458.1.

"Paul J. Arciero." Paul Arciero. Accessed November 24, 2017. https://www.skidmore. edu/ exercisescience/faculty/paul-arciero.php.

Palmore, Erdman B., Frank Whittington, and Suzanne Kunkel, eds. The International Handbook on Aging: Current Research and Developments. 3rd ed. Santa Barbara, CA: Praeger, 2009.

Park, Sung Kyun, Joel Schwartz, Marc Weisskopf, David Sparrow, Pantel S. Vokonas,

"Pete Seeger—Keep Your Eyes on the Prize." Genius. Accessed February 16, 2018. https:// genius.com/Pete-seeger-keep-your-eyes-on-the-prize-lyrics.

Pogue, David. "Fitness Trackers Are Everywhere, but Do They Work?" Scientific American.

January 01, 2015. Accessed March 2, 2018. https://www.scientificamerican.com/ article/ fitness-trackers-are-everywhere-but-do-they-work/.

"PsycNET." American Psychological Association. Accessed January 8, 2018. http:// psycnet. apa.org/record/1975-26412-001.

Quantum Emergence System | Dr Matt Mannino. Accessed March 3, 2018. http:// quantumemergence.com/qe/.

"Recent Perspectives Regarding the Role of Dietary Protein for the Promotion of Muscle Hypertrophy with Resistance Exercise Training." Nutrients 10, no. 2 (2018): 180. doi:10.3390/nu10020180.

Rice, Xan. "Rise of the Super-Agers: As the 100-Year Life Becomes More Common, the Exploits of an Extraordinary Set of Athletes Are Forcing Scientists to Reassess the Relationship between Performance and Growing Old." New Statesman (1996), April 7, 2017, 46+.

Robert O. Wright, Brent Coull, Huiling Nie, and Howard Hu. "Low-Level Lead Exposure, Metabolic Syndrome, and Heart Rate Variability: The VA Normative Aging Study." Environmental Health Perspectives 114, no. 11 (2006): 1718+.

Rognmo, O., T. Moholdt, H. Bakken, T. Hole, P. Molstad, N. E. Myhr, J. Grimsmo, and U. Wisloff. "Cardiovascular Risk of High-Versus Moderate-Intensity Aerobic Exercise in Coronary Heart Disease Patients." Circulation 126, no. 12 (2012): 1436-440. doi:10.1161/circulationaha.112.123117.

Roos, V.; Ronn, M.; Salihovic, S.; Lind, L.; van Bavel, B.; Kullberg, J.; Johansson, L.; Ahlstrom, H.; Lind, P.M. "Circulating levels of persistent organic pollutants in relation to visceral and subcutaneous adipose tissue by abdominal MRI." Obesity 2013, 21, 413–418.

Ross, Benjamin, and Steven Amter. The Polluters: The Making of Our Chemically-Altered Environment. New York: Oxford University Press, 2010.

Rothblum, Esther, and Sondra Solovay, eds. The Fat Studies Reader. New York: New York University Press, 2009.

Ruby M, Repka CP, Arciero PJ. "Comparison of Protein-Pacing Alone or With Yoga/ Stretching and Resistance Training on Glycemia, Total and Regional Body Composition, and Aerobic Fitness in Overweight Women." J Phys Act Health. 2016 Jul;13(7):754-64

Salvi, Kristin. "Paul Arciero, New York." You're the Cure. Accessed March 10, 2018. https:// www.yourethecure.org/paul_arciero_new_york.

"Samples.jbpub.com." Jbpub. Accessed January 8, 2018. http://samples.jbpub. com./9781284034851/Chapter_3.pdf.

ScienceDaily. Accessed November 22, 2017. https://www.sciencedaily.com/ releases/2017/01/170111184102.htm.

Scutti, Susan. "A Gut Reaction." Newsweek, November 29, 2013.

"Selected Issues for Nutrition and the Athlete: A Team...:Medicine & Science in Sports & Exercise." LWW. Accessed February 2, 2018. https://journals.lww. com/acsm-msse/ Fulltext/2013/12000/Selected_Issues_for_Nutrition_and_ the_Athlete_A.21.aspx.

Shahzad, Mian M. K., Mildred Felder, Kai Ludwig, Hannah R. Van Galder, Matthew L. Anderson, Jong Kim, Mark E. Cook, Arvinder K. Kapur, and Manish S. Patankar. "Trans10,cis12 conjugated linoleic acid inhibits proliferation and migration of ovarian cancer cells by inducing ER stress, autophagy, and modulation of Src." PLOS ONE. January 11, 2018. Accessed February 23, 2018. http://paperity.org/p/85521415/ trans10-cis12-conjugated-linoleic-acid-inhibits-proliferation-and-migration-of-ovarian.

Shearrer, GE, MJ. Daniels, CM. Toledo-Corral, MJ. Weigensberg, D. Spruijt-Metz, and JN. Davis. "Associations among sugar sweetened beverage intake, visceral fat, and cortisol awakening response in minority youth." Physiology & Behavior 167 (2016): 188-93. doi:10.1016/j.physbeh.2016.09.020.

"Six Yoga Exercises That Could Change Your Life; Your Life Daily EVERYONE Loves A Quick Fix—Whether It Is to Perfect Your Face, Achieve a Body Beautiful or Whittle Down That Weight. So Wouldn't It Be Great to Be Able to Do Just a Few Simple Exercises a Day to Boost the Body, Mind, and Soul? KAREN HAMBRIDGE Investigates. New Year New You." Coventry Evening Telegraph (England), January 14, 2008.

Skibola, Christine F., Jianqing Zhang, and Jacques E. Riby. "Heavy Metal Contamination of Powdered Protein and Botanical Shake Mixes." Journal of Environmental Health 80, no. 4 (2017): 8+.

"Skidmore and local school students mark National Eating Healthy Day." The Saratogian. November 07, 2012. Accessed March 10, 2018. http://www. saratogian.com/article/ ST/20121107/NEWS/311079911.

"Skidmore professor headed to Washington to talk about health." NEWS10 ABC. May 11, 2015. Accessed March 10, 2018. http://news10.com/2015/05/10/ skidmore-professor-headed-to-washington-to-talk-about-health/.

Skidmore College. "Diet helps shed pounds, release toxins and reduce oxidative stress." ScienceDaily. ScienceDaily, 11 January 2017. Available at: www.sciencedaily.com/ releases/2017/01/170111184102.htm.

"Statistics About Diabetes." American Diabetes Association. Accessed February 23, 2018. http://www.diabetes.org/diabetes-basics/statistics/.

"Stephen F. Austin State University." Kinesiology and Health Science | SFASU. Accessed February 22, 2018. http://www.sfasu.edu/kinesiology.

Streeter, Chris C., Theodore H. Whitfield, Liz Owen, Tasha Rein, Surya K. Karri, Aleksandra Yakhkind, Ruth Perlmutter, Andrew Prescot, Perry F. Renshaw, Domenic A. Ciraulo, and J. Eric Jensen. Journal of Alternative and Complementary Medicine. November 2010.

Accessed March 20, 2018. https://www.ncbi.nlm.nih.gov/pmc/articles/PMC3111147/.

Taubes, Gary. "What if It's All Been a Big Fat Lie?" The New York Times. July 07, 2002.

Accessed February 14, 2018. http://www.nytimes.com/2002/07/07/magazine/what-if-it-s-all-been-a-big-fat-lie.html?pagewanted=1.

"The Carnegie Classification of Institutions of Higher Education." Carnegie Classifications|Listings. Accessed January 8, 2018. http://carnegieclassifications. iu.edu/

listings.php.

"Try These Four Ways to Slow Down the Ageing Process; Take Control of Your Chronological Age." Coffs Coast Advocate (Coffs Harbour, Australia), February 28, 2015.

Ungar, Peter S., and Mark F. Teaford, eds. Human Diet: Its Origin and Evolution. Westport, CT: Bergin and Garvey, 2002.

"US Data & Trends Redirect." Centers for Disease Control and Prevention. April 04, 2012. Accessed February 23, 2018. https://www.cdc.gov/diabetes/statistics/slides/long_ term_trends.pdf .

Valeria, Rosato, Valentina, Maria, Gabriella, Lorenzo, Emilio, Monica, Decarli, and Adriano. "Effect of breakfast composition and energy contribution on cognitive and academic performance: a systematic review | The American Journal of Clinical Nutrition | Oxford Academic." OUP Academic. May 27, 2014. Accessed March 8, 2018. https://academic. oup.com/ajcn/article/100/2/626/4576549.

"Vital: 20 FOODS TO BOOST YOUR ENERGY." Daily Record (Glasgow, Scotland), May 17, 2005.

Walford, Roy L. Beyond the 120-Year Diet: How to Double Your Vital Years. Revised ed. New York: Four Walls Eight Windows, 2000.

Wang, Duolao, and Ameet Bakhai. Clinical trials: a practical guide to design, analysis, and reporting. London: Remedica, 2006.

"Want to Lose Weight? Boost Gut Health for Effective Results." Hindustan Times (New Delhi, India), April 23, 2016.

Waterhouse, J., G. Atkinson, B. Edwards, and T. Reilly. "The role of a short post-lunch nap in improving cognitive, motor, and sprint performance in participants with partial sleep deprivation." Journal of Sports Sciences. December 2007. Accessed March 15, 2018. https://www.ncbi.nlm.nih.gov/pubmed/17852691.

Weston, Kassia S., Ulrik Wisløff, and Jeff S. Coombes. "High-intensity interval training in patients with lifestyle-induced cardiometabolic disease: a systematic review and meta- analysis." British Journal of Sports Medicine 48, no. 16 (2013): 1227-234. doi:10.1136/ bjsports-2013-092576.

"What Is BPA? Should I Be Worried About It?—Mayo Clinic." 2017. Mayo Clinic. http:// www.mayoclinic.org/healthy-lifestyle/nutrition-and-healthy-eating/ expert-answers/ bpa/faq-20058331

Whoriskey, Peter. "The science of skipping breakfast: How government nutritionists may have gotten it wrong." The Washington Post. August 10, 2015. Accessed March 18, 2018. https://www.washingtonpost.com/news/wonk/wp/2015/08/10/ the-science-of- skipping-breakfast-how-government-nutritionists-may-have-gotten-it-wrong/?utm_ term=.60d3aca497fa.

"Why We Got Fatter During The Fat-Free Food Boom." 2017. NPR.Org. http://www. npr.org/ sections/thesalt/2014/03/28/295332576/ why-we-got-fatter-during-the-fat-free-food-boom

"World Health Organization Assesses the World's Health Systems." WHO. Accessed January 8, 2018. http://www.who.int/whr/2000/media_centre/press_release/ en/.

"You Can Now Snort Chocolate, But Doctors Aren't Happy About It." Health. com. Accessed March 10, 2018. http://www.health.com/nutrition/snortable-chocolate-coco-loko.

"Your Health." Daily Herald (Arlington Heights, IL), February 13, 2017.

Zohar, Sarah. "Phase I/II Clinical Trials." Methods and Applications of Statistics in Clinical Trials, 2014, 658-66. doi:10.1002/9781118596005.ch54.

Zuo, Li, Feng He, Grant M. Tinsley, Benjamin K. Pannell, Emery Ward, and Paul J. Arciero. "Comparison of High-Protein, Intermittent Fasting Low-Calorie Diet and Heart Healthy Diet for Vascular Health of the Obese." Frontiers in Physiology 7 (2016). doi:10.3389/ fphys.2016.00350.

ACCOLADES

THE RESEARCH: STATS ON DR. PAUL

Advisory Board Positions
International Protein Board (IPB, www.internationalproteinboard.com)

American Heart Association (Capital Region)

Dymatize Nutrition

Isagenix International LLC

Fellow
The Obesity Society (FTOS)

American College of Sports Medicine (FACSM)

International Society of Sports Nutrition (FISSN)

Nutrition Consultant
Isagenix International

Abbott Nutrition, EAS

Dymatize

*Consultant for:
United States Army - Special Operation Forces (Green Berets)

Olympic Medalists

National Hockey League and American Hockey League

Thousands of master's, NCAA collegiate and high school athletes

*Studies Published in:

American Journal of Preventive Medicine

Journal of Clinical Medicine

Frontiers in Aging Neuroscience

Frontiers in Physiology

American Journal of Physiology

Journal of Applied Physiology

American Journal of Clinical Nutrition

Journal of the International Neuropsychological Society

Frontiers in Human Neuroscience

*See Dr. Paul in these Publications and Media Outlets:

O Magazine	Huffington Post	Muscle and Fitness
The Wall Street	Daily Mail	Men's Fitness
Journal	SELF	Men's Health
Fox News	Glamour	Doctor Radio - XM/
Prevention	Shape	Sirius
Good Housekeeping	Health	National Public Radio
WebMD	Women's Health	
TIME	Women's World	

*For a full list please visit www.paularciero.com/accolades

ABOUT THE AUTHOR

Paul Arciero, PhD, FACSM, FTOS, FISSN, is a leading international nutrition and applied physiology scientist and researcher, professor, keynote speaker, consultant, world-class athlete and Amazon No. 1 bestselling author. He earned a masters of science in nutrition from the University of Vermont School of Medicine and Nutritional Sciences, as well as a masters of science in exercise physiology from Purdue University. He earned a doctorate in exercise physiology from Springfield College, and held a postdoctoral fellowship in applied physiology from Washington University School of Medicine.

Since 1994, Dr. Paul has been a professor (full professor since 2010) in the Department of Health and Human Physiological Sciences, and the director of the Human Nutrition, Metabolism and Performance Laboratory at Skidmore College in Saratoga Springs, NY. He is also a research professor in the Psychology and Neurosciences Department at Union College in Schenectady, NY.

With more than thirty years of dedicated science-based research, Dr. Paul has over sixty peer-reviewed published scientific articles, and is considered a go-to content expert by the highest level media outlets. He is the pioneer and leading expert on teaching how to use Protein Pacing, The PRISE Life Protocol, and The PRISE Life app to help you live the "PRISE Life"!

Dr. Paul is also a European tennis champion, former top-ranked NCAA tennis player, and NCAA head tennis coach, Empire State Games gold and silver medalist, and multiple-time triathlon and road running race winner. He offers consulting services for nutrition, fitness and wellness and his speeches draw audiences into the tens of thousands. His devotion to helping people achieve optimal health and peak performance—from star athletes to the already overstressed busy person—is contagious.

Join Dr. Paul to live a life of optimum health and peak performance! Please visit www.priselife.com for more information. To book Dr. Paul as your next keynote speaker visit www.paularciero.com.

www.ingramcontent.com/pod-product-compliance
Lightning Source LLC
Chambersburg PA
CBHW060315030426
42336CB00011B/1057